Chastened

Hephzibah Anderson

Chastened

THE UNEXPECTED STORY
OF MY YEAR WITHOUT SEX

VIKING

VIKING
Published by the Penguin Group
Penguin Group (USA) Inc., 375 Hudson Street, New York, New York 10014, U.S.A.
Penguin Group (Canada), 90 Eglinton Avenue East, Suite 700, Toronto, Ontario, Canada M4P 2Y3
(a division of Pearson Penguin Canada Inc.)   ·   Penguin Books Ltd, 80 Strand, London WC2R 0RL,
England   ·   Penguin Ireland, 25 St. Stephen's Green, Dublin 2, Ireland (a division of Penguin Books Ltd)
Penguin Books Australia Ltd, 250 Camberwell Road, Camberwell, Victoria 3124, Australia (a division
of Pearson Australia Group Pty Ltd)   ·   Penguin Books India Pvt Ltd, 11 Community Centre,
Panchsheel Park, New Delhi – 110 017, India   ·   Penguin Group (NZ), 67 Apollo Drive, Rosedale,
North Shore 0632, New Zealand (a division of Pearson New Zealand Ltd)   ·   Penguin Books (South
Africa) (Pty) Ltd, 24 Sturdee Avenue, Rosebank, Johannesburg 2196, South Africa

Penguin Books Ltd, Registered Offices: 80 Strand, London WC2R 0RL, England

First American edition
Published in 2010 by Viking Penguin, a member of Penguin Group (USA) Inc.

1   3   5   7   9   10   8   6   4   2

Copyright © Hephzibah Anderson, 2009, 2010
All rights reserved

Excerpt from "We Didn't" from *I Sailed with Magellan* by Stuart Dybek (Farrar, Straus and Giroux).
Copyright © 2003 by Stuart Dybek.   ·   Excerpt from *The Female Eunuch* by Germaine Greer
(HarperCollins). Copyright © 1970, 1971 by Germaine Greer   ·   Excerpt from "Hilda and Rongo" from
Little Birds by Anaïs Nin (Harcourt). Copyright © 1979 by Rupert Pole as Trustee under the Last Will and
Testament of Anaïs Nin. By permission of Barbara W. Stuhlmann, author's representative.   ·   Excerpt
from *The Change* by Germaine Greer (Alfred A. Knopf). Copyright © 1991 by Germaine Greer.

LIBRARY OF CONGRESS CATALOGING IN PUBLICATION DATA
Anderson, Hephzibah.
Chastened : the unexpected story of my year without sex / Hephzibah Anderson.
p. cm.
"First published in Great Britain in 2009 by Chatto & Windus"—T.p. verso.
ISBN 978-0-670-02186-4
1. Anderson, Hephzibah—Sexual behavior. 2. Anderson, Hephzibah—Relations with men. 3. Sexual
abstinence—United States—Case studies. 4. Chastity—Case studies. 5. Women—Sexual behavior—
United States—Case studies. 6. Man-woman relationships—United States—Case studies. 7. Single
women—New York (State)—New York—Biography. 8. New York (N.Y.)—Biography. I. Title.
HQ29.A495 2009
306.73'2092—dc22 [B]   2009047240

Printed in the United States of America
Set in Arrus   ·   Designed by Amy Hill

*Penguin is committed to publishing works of quality and integrity.
In that spirit, we are proud to offer this book to our readers;
however, the story, the experiences, and the words
are the author's alone.*

For my mother,
who should probably read no further,
and my sister, who knows it all without having to

We didn't in the light; we didn't in darkness. We didn't in the fresh-cut summer grass or in the mounds of autumn leaves or on the snow where moonlight threw down our shadows.

—Stuart Dybek, "We Didn't"

Contents

Introduction

MIRANDA: I can't have dinner with you;
I don't even know you!

BARTENDER: But you slept with me!

MIRANDA: That's a different thing.

—*Sex and the City*

When you decide to give up sex and begin a year of chastity, it's not something you rush to tell people. In a supersexualized society that uses orgasms to sell shampoo and produces pole-dancing kits for kids, in which a sensual account of brother-sister incest goes unremarked upon in a respected broadsheet and even online avatars are having affairs, opting out feels like the last conceivable taboo. In my own case, I'd assumed I was retreating into a more private sphere. It never occurred to me to blog about my quest, and the book you are holding in your hands was an idea that arrived late in the journey. For a while, I didn't tell my friends, either. When I did tentatively step out of my chaste closet, I found that others didn't quite see it the same way. In fact, they felt licensed to ask all sorts of questions that they'd ordinarily have kept to themselves.

"What do you *do*?" wondered one girl, squinting at me in disbelief. "Masturbation—is that allowed?" an older male friend wanted to know, leaning closer and flashing a red-wine grin. "Is it because of me?" asked a guy who'd once invited me home with him (I hadn't taken him up on the offer, but maybe he was muddling me up with a girl who had). And then there was the question that came up most often—what did I have planned for my year's end? As an ex put it, "There has to be some kind of payoff, right?" If there was going to be a party, nobody wanted to miss it.

The question I heard least frequently was the only one I'd really been anticipating: why? Plenty of people, I would realize, have thought about hopping off the sexual merry-go-round. Sex and its pursuit seem to have become such blood sports, their rules so confusing and their standards so exacting, that it is hard not to wonder occasionally whether it's worth it. At the same time, sexiness is so ubiquitous, it has become a bit of a turnoff. In the past decade, everything from political dossiers to ballroom dancing has been "sexed up." You needn't even be getting any to feel jaded, and that's perhaps part of the problem: it's not so much sex that's everywhere, but a toned, tanned, airbrushed pastiche that verges on neutering and has less and less to do with the real thing.

I'd thought those thoughts once or twice, but it would never have occurred to me that I'd actually go ahead and voluntarily eject sex from my life. It took a bizarre serendipity, a torrid affair and a chance anecdote to make me realize that the kind of sex I was supposed to be cool with as a postfeminist, twenty-first-century Western woman—a casual sort of intimacy without intimacy—was not working for me. To explain fully, I need to beckon you back in time to a sunny afternoon in New York City. But first, those other questions.

What do I do? It turns out that there is much that doesn't involve sex. It is impossible for a human being to endure more than three days without water. With water but no food, you might make it to three weeks. Shelter and warmth are additional necessities, sunlight a boon, and peace and love will ease your years. But one thing not remotely essential is sex, though you'd never guess it from the material that bombards you whenever you switch on the telly, flip through a magazine or delete another screenful of spam. All right, in most circumstances it's still just about required for life's perpetuation, but we can lead perfectly healthy and, indeed, happy existences without nooky, whoopee or bonking. People can—and do—go decades without sex. Some live their entire lives without it.

While the birds and the bees and the penguins on the rocks are busy doing it, nuns, mystics and athletes-in-training have found plenty else to be getting on with, and they aren't the only ones. Elizabeth I was known as the Virgin Queen, and there was nothing metaphorical about the title, history assures us. Gandhi became celibate at age thirty-six, despite still being married. (What his wife thought of this—or of his late-life decision to test his resolve by sharing his bed with a procession of nubile young girls—is not recorded.) The Shakers even founded a faith based around chastity. Interviewed on the eve of her 105th birthday in October 2008, Cornwall resident Clara Meadmore attributed her longevity to having remained a virgin. On the subject of relationships, she added, "I imagine there is a lot of hassle involved and I have always been busy doing other things."

But I don't think this was what my friend had in mind when she asked me what I *did*. Where did I draw the line, she meant, which segues neatly into that second question: was I intending to pass up *all* sexual pleasure? One of my motivations for embracing chastity was a sense that sex had grown impersonal—that it was nothing more than a game of tennis, as a thirtysomething marketing whiz insisted to me while I was researching a magazine article on casual sex. More than what he'd said, it was his tone that got me: matter-of-fact, without any frisson of joy. He wasn't even trying to shock.

I've never been any good at tennis, whether on grass, clay or high-thread-count Egyptian cotton. Yet I felt like I was the one at fault, so I kept trying. Sometimes my decision to have sex seemed to be based more on what was appropriate to the moment than on what was right for me. At a certain point in certain scenarios, a part of me abdicated and gave in to the inevitable. Tipsily noticing that it was after midnight and I was far from home, say, in a dwindling group that happened to include a man I'd found myself in bed with some-time before. "That was intense," he'd said afterward, as if intensity were something unexpected in sex. But it was intense, and which-ever bit of me had abdicated, it was never my heart. Wouldn't it be fun to have sex that was purely, deliciously physical? It would cer-tainly smooth some of the more tempestuous aspects of dating, but at the same time I secretly dreaded that I might finally get the hang of bedroom tennis. Once you've learned to separate sex from emo-tion, how simple is it to put them back together?

So when it came to making rules for my experiment, they were unabashedly personal. What I'd discovered was that I could deal with any amount of orgasmic foreplay along the way, but it was last base—what sex-ed instructors brave sniggers to term penile pene-tration—that tipped me over the edge. I had given something of myself, and accordingly, that was the moment at which I started needing more than I might ever have wanted from the man in ques-tion, the moment he went in my eyes from being an unassuming frog to being a shiny prince.

It seemed illogical—possibly also biological, psychological, socio-logical. And yes, it had to do with numbers as well—those tallies we each carry around with us, inscribed in our minds (because they don't always belong in our hearts) in the faintest pencil lest anyone see them. Mine is a greater number than I'd like and contains some names I'd rather forget. I won't tell you exactly what it is, because a note of coyness here seems more instructive: while we're no longer supposed to be judged for our sexual conduct, we all know that the double standard lingers on. Even if men have got over it, we women have not. A tiny bit of me can't help judging myself, nor, presum-ably, can those women who consistently shave their own tallies in sex surveys. Perhaps it's just that we know that not every one of those strikes is without regret; that as we count them off, we pause over this one or that, recalling how the fun was seasoned with some-thing that made us feel less good about ourselves. Liberated women that we are, we'll blame Victorian morality and its outmoded, re-pressive mores—we'll blame ourselves for succumbing and we'll deny our feelings. Because penile-penetrative sex is what it took for me to add to that list, it was also where I drew my line. (And put in such blunt terms—well, it didn't sound all that desirable anyway.)

Though definitions differ among gays and lesbians, an over-whelming number of heterosexuals continue to view that moment as the moment a person loses their virginity. I wasn't rushing to join those women who declared themselves "revirginized," either figura-tively or literally (yes, literally—it's called vaginoplasty), but I did badly want sex to be legitimately momentous again, rather than an inexorable conclusion given the right cocktail of time and place, as had begun to seem the case. I wanted to revel in the intensity of it all, to believe in the meaning that my body gave the experience, with-out worrying about when or even whether he'd call, and without feeling like a failure for letting the thought cloud the moment. That, I suppose, was the payoff I was ultimately craving—that in our newly thrifty times, chastity would not only remind me of the erotic rewards of delayed gratification but would return me to a place where I could feel I was being faithful to my own instincts.

Later, I'd learn that others before me had incorporated the same working definition into their own chaste regimens, but I didn't know this when I set off on my journey, and I'm glad: it made my quest more private, and the very idea of privacy is enticingly subversive. While social networking facilities like Facebook and Twitter encourage us to make public our most trivial triumphs and fleeting frustrations, from the sandwich we ate for lunch to the soaking we got on our way back to the office, multifunctional gadgets enable us to fill what might once have been moments of enforced contemplation with the chatter of texts and e-mails, iTunes and YouTube clips. Our diminishing sense of privacy and of a hidden internal space seems to have robbed sex of something thrilling.

My only other rule was that my year would start not from the time I last had sex but from the day I made my decision. After all, I'm certain I've had dry spells that lasted longer than twelve months. It was the choosing that was crucial, even if it meant adding another three weeks to my challenge. Rather than continuing to go along with what others seemed to want from sex, I had to rediscover what it meant to me. Most urgently, I had to find my way back to the place where love and sex intersected for real. Making that initial decision seemed like a step in the right direction.

Oh, but I know what you're thinking. You're thinking, "A year without sex? Well, what's the big deal? Many are the times *I've* gone that long—longer—without." Or maybe just, "How vain! What, she reckons she's so irresistible she'll be fighting them off? Such a tease, such a tramp, such a hussy!" Because after all, you'd think a challenge or two would be necessary to make it a valid experiment. Then again, perhaps you suspect I'm judging you. "Hang on," you're thinking. "Who's she to call *me* a hussy? So she's had her fun and now she's trying to tell *us* how to behave?" I'm not, incidentally, though there are plenty of competing views out there on how we should conduct our most intimate affairs, and when I embarked upon my quest, I knew that I'd have to negotiate them along the way.

We may stroll blithely past a sex-toy shop or casually add the latest call-girl memoir to our three-for-two pile in the bookshop, but despite its presentation as just another recreational activity, sex is still a subject that we take deeply personally. Even in the abstract, there's nothing quite like it for getting the heart pumping and making ordinarily rational people prickly, pugnacious, downright irrational. A couple of days after that feature on casual sex appeared, I ran into a colleague. "You ruined my weekend," she said, only partly joking. "I spent a whole day feeling bad because all those people you interviewed are having all that sex and I'm not. And I'm actually in a relationship," she added, as if the contradiction had only just struck her.

Then again, perhaps you're not thinking any of this; perhaps you're muttering just one word: "*Cheat.*" After all, foreplay can be vastly more satisfying than what follows. At other times, merely falling asleep beside someone—dreaming together and waking together—is a far more intimate experience than *sleeping* with them in the coyer sense. Those who go in for giving up sex are gluttons for nothing if not deprivation. John Harvey Kellogg, for instance, eschewed a long list of additional activities, including waltzing and the consumption of rich foods (the cornflakes that tumble into your bowl each morning were originally part of a plan far more ambitious than a quick, healthy breakfast). St. Simeon the Stylite, a shepherd's son born at the end of the fourth century, lived into his sixties at the top of a sixty-foot-high pillar. While he ascended to abstemious asceticism up above, he permitted male pilgrims to gather below. All women, including his mother, were banned. And yet here I am, giving up sex for a mere twelve months, while still allowing myself to indulge in rich foods, high heels and bright society, not to mention the thrill of the chase. Where is the challenge in that? you may wonder.

But here is my point: unlike the nuns whose flowing habits epitomize chastity, I had no desire to deny my sexuality, and nor was the experiment ever meant to be about withdrawing from intimacy. All I was giving up was sex. I'd turned thirty a few months before taking my vow, and, among other things, was looking for a fresh way of pursuing love into that new decade—a way that was a little less ungainly, permitted a little more self-respect and might even yield a little more success. In that regard, adopting an unrealistically nunnish definition would not have helped. There is also this: after almost a decade of ricocheting from one short-lived romantic fiasco to another, I'd forgotten that the chase could be fun.

While sex is everywhere, it's only when you've sworn off that you really begin to notice. It's in the swing of a cute waiter's hips, the tilt of a head and the gaze you know you shouldn't hold—certainly not for this long. It's very definitely in the roaming hands of a date—your lucky third—with that man whose new apartment is fortunately still missing a sofa, because sofas positively sigh sex. It's in the ellipsis at the end of a text message sealed with a tantalizing single kiss. It's in the song whose lyrics won't quit bumping and grinding in your head—the one that begins with a guy asking a girl how many times a night she needs "it." More troublingly, it's in the slogans that decorate T-shirts for preteens, and in the thrusting postures of cartoon women decorating checkout chocolate bars. It's in the name of the red nail polish—Temptress—that you pick out on a blue day.

A year, it turns out, can feel like a very long time indeed, and though I didn't know it back when I was drawing up my rules, in allowing myself all the good things that lead up to sex, I was unwittingly making the challenge infinitely harder. But all that comes later. For now, I need to take you back to the very start—to the bizarre serendipity that preceded the torrid affair and the chance anecdote, to the glimpse of a path not taken, which set me on this unexpected journey.

Chastened

ONE

My First Time

Nobody dies from lack of sex.
It's lack of love we die from.

—Margaret Atwood,
The Handmaid's Tale

The backdrop is Manhattan, still summer-warm despite the early-October date. I'm travel-dazed after a late-night scramble to clear my desk and pack my bags, tumbling into a cab and through the damp London dawn to the airport. The driver chatted in an accent that was impossible to place but audibly distant, casting us adrift as we coasted through familiar streets made foreign by their emptiness. Was I traveling for business or pleasure? he asked. Both, I replied, unable to recall when the distinction grew so blurred.

Having landed at noon and muddled through an accommodation mix-up and a meeting, I'm now trying to reorient myself, letting my feet remember the island's east and west, its uptown and downtown, a topography so simple it can be baffling. This must be how I end up on Fifth Avenue, borne along by the ceaseless flow of pedestrian traffic. Already the sun is dipping in the sky, bouncing off the city's silvered pillars and sending slices of itself skittering into infinity. It's bedazzling, and bedazzled, I pause at a crossing, teetering on the curb, my eyes trained on the faces of the crowd opposite, waiting for the surge to carry me over.

It's then that I see him: Dan, my university boyfriend, my first.

It's not that he looks exactly as I remember him. He has thinned and thickened a little in all the wrong places, but something in his physical presence—a way of advancing through the world—triggers a jolt of recognition in the eye-blink moment of his passing. Muscle memory is the strongest, a dance teacher once told me, and as I stand here on Fifth Avenue, which is yellow with cabs loudly going nowhere, I can't help but fancifully wonder whether that oughtn't make the heart's memories clearest of all, because some small portion of mine still knows the boy who claimed it all those years ago.

Oh, how I'd adored him! He'd been smart and stormily good-looking, animated by a kind of reckless energy that kept his shoulders as tense as a boxer's. His smile had a broken edge to it, hinting at just the right amount of vulnerability. We'd met toward the end of the second year at university, at what, with youth's exhausting irony, we called a "bop," this particular one celebrating the kitschiness of the Eurovision Song Contest. It was 1996, and the United Kingdom's losing entry, "Ooh Ahh . . . Just a Little Bit" by Gina G, was about to become our song.

Dan's winning flaw was his klutziness. If ever anything was going to be dropped—especially something involving clatter and mess—it would fall from his hands. He was the same on the dance floor—not a bad dancer, just all over the place, jostling me with his elbows and feet. Each time, he'd apologize. Each time, our smiles grew a little more beaming, our eye contact a little longer lasting.

Later, as the lights came mercilessly up on a roomful of party-smeared faces, our friends sloped off to join the coat queue while we chatted—or didn't, not really, because it seemed as if something had already been agreed upon, so what more was there to say? But I must have told him my name and where to find me, because a few days later, a note appeared in my college pigeonhole, asking if I'd like to meet for a drink. Back then, there was no choice but to be romantic. Today that note would be a text or an e-mail—thrilling in its way yet not nearly as intimate as handwriting, with its cryptic quirks and flaws. The text lives only on your SIM card; the e-mail may be printed off a hundred times in a few keystrokes, which perhaps explains why we so seldom bother to print it even once. But the note, with its tactile permeability, can be kept, loved, lost.

You should know that the Eurovision meeting wasn't technically our first. That had occurred almost two years before. I'd tagged along to a welcome-week mixer and been introduced by a school friend of his. We didn't talk much. The friend was flirty and wise-cracking, but Dan had a heavier presence, quarrelsome and sulky-seeming. Months and months passed before a girl breathlessly pointed him out to me at some other sticky-floored party. Taking a second look, I saw that that dark cloud of a boy had grown glossy. His inky eyes gleamed, making any lingering antagonism seem like an appealing challenge.

Many years later, sitting in a cheap restaurant in Paris on a cool spring night, a girlfriend would share a favorite saying with me: "He chased her until she caught him." Thinking back to that distant moment when I followed another girl's gaze through the student fug, I'd smile, knowing that on that night, my trap was set. I've grown less sure of my own judgment since.

We soon became inseparable. Fine weather arrived early that year, and we'd meet after exams to lie stretched out on the riverbank as dusk fell, sharp and earthy. Drunk with the joy of it all, I forgot to eat and grew skinny on romance. I daydreamed and became the girl I'd always scorned, abandoning my friends for nights out with his. When the term ended, we enmeshed ourselves in each other's families. We'd both won salaried work placements and spent the summer playing at being adults, he in a suit, I in heels, joining the crowds outside city pubs on fine evenings. He left shirts at my place. My panties found their way under his bed. One night, I sat watching him cook. He had lovely hands, and there was nothing clumsy about him as he darted between the stove and the fridge, stirring this, dicing that, pausing to offer a taste. This is how I want my life to be when I grow up, I thought, leaning into the jacket he'd slung over the back of my chair and breathing him in with the scent of dinner.

Later on that summer, we traveled together, driving through deserts and picnicking on the hot hood of a rental car—fiery pickles to cut through the oily dips, a chocolate drink from childhood, greedy mouthfuls of warm beer to wash it all down with. Our kisses were salty-sweet with a hint of suntan lotion, and at night we lay naked while creaking ceiling fans churned the muggy air of one budget room after another. We got lost, capsized kayaks, almost drove straight across a divided highway—somehow it didn't matter. Something solidified between us during that trip.

We were in Israel for the Yom Kippur fast, sat beside Lake Kinneret in the green north as the country wound down. All was quiet save for the gentle slap and swoosh of waves against the side of a moored party boat—the kind that sails in circles for birthdays and weddings—and the soft sound of reggae drifting from belowdecks, smudging the warm night air. Across the water, lights shimmered on the far shore, but above and before us lay only expanses of liquid, star-spattered nothing. We talked a lot that night, sipping beers cadged from one of the dreadlocked men onboard, but our silences said just as much as we peered ahead together to the coming academic year—our last—and beyond.

With the new term, we settled precociously into snug domesticity. During our entire third year, we spent just one night apart. Somewhere in a shoebox of jumbled snaps is a picture of the two of us at a garden party shortly before graduation. We're dolled up like a pair of dandies, his arm encircling my waist, a cigarette and champagne for props. Heavy-headed blooms fill out the shot, lending it the air of an old-fashioned wedding portrait, though looking at it after all these years, I'd say it's our purposefulness, our certainty, that seems most striking, eclipsing even our youth.

Finals were sat, graduation came and went and suddenly we were leaving.

"Don't look back," Dan told me as we drove into the future. And I didn't, not then, nor the morning a few months later when I woke to the realization that I was no longer in love with him. Not until that sun-struck New York afternoon eight years later do I glance back. This is what I see: my university boyfriend, my first, walking away with his arm slung over the shoulders of another girl. She's petite and honey-haired, and he's steering her into a store.

Into De Beers.

It's a scenario that could have been plucked straight from one of the novels that come my way as a book critic, or, more likely, from one of the films that I gulp down so indiscriminately in my spare time. If our sidewalk scene really had been fiction, I'd have called out, Dan would have turned, and in the same instant we'd both have been struck by the gleaming knowledge that we were meant to be together, blissfully ever after, leaving the small blonde to melt away into a comic subplot. In fact, the episode's sheer unreality kept my lips sealed, but it didn't guard me from its spell.

Later on during that same visit, I strayed into a museum gift shop, and among the pencils and key fobs found a fat ring made of clear Perspex—like a miniature snow globe, except that its vacant half-sphere was filled with glitter. A silver-haired assistant saw me shaking up a blizzard of sparkle and smiled as I tried to wriggle it off my finger.

"I'd have loved this when I was little," I said, embarrassed. I loved it at age twenty-nine and three-quarters, and she knew it.

"Everyone needs a bit of magic in their lives," she told me. It should have sounded hokey, except that she rang it up on the till with such pleasing matter-of-factness.

We twenty-first-century atheists and agnostics place so much faith in love. We scan horoscopes for it and credit it with all sorts of transformative powers. We become passive before its might, waiting for it to happen to us, and when it does, we duly drop to our knees and marvel at the power that guided us to it through life's maze of chance and happenstance. That New York glimpse of first love felt important, and it was enough to get me thinking. Call it coincidence, call it fate—call it, if you prefer to, a snatched-at half-sighting of something that was or perhaps was not. For me, the very fact that I *thought* I'd seen Dan was amply significant. Back in London, the city we both called home, I'd run into him just once, half a dozen years before, yet here he seemingly was. Hallucinating ex-boyfriends, this was where my giddy, lovelorn twenties had ditched me.

And why would Dan not have been holding the De Beers door open for *me?* you might be wondering. From almost a decade's distance, that relationship seems both unattainably simple and undesirably simplistic. We were so struck with each other that our togetherness felt like play—the serious, hard play that gets forgotten in adulthood. Yes, there was plenty wrong with it—my jilted friends thought I was too in thrall to him, and the two of us dodged important conversations—yet those faults never seemed a match for whatever it was that bound us together. Was it sex? I think maybe it was, but that isn't to say it was *just* sex. That kind of sex was something I'd yet to encounter, because here's the thing: Dan was the boy I lost my virginity to.

Given our time and place—the anything-goes West at the tail end of the seen-it-all twentieth century—I was a very late starter. I was twenty, which made me around four years older than the UK's national average as it then was, almost a spinster by panicky post-adolescent standards. At school, an invisible divide had begun opening up from the age of fifteen or so between those of us who'd "done it" and the rest of us, who'd only read about it in well-thumbed Judy Blume and Sweet Valley High books. One of my closest friends crossed over and went through a moody, withdrawn phase, losing an alarming amount of weight as she spent lunch hours sitting in the lap of her straggly-haired lover.

Senior year at high school was self-selectingly nerdy, so even at seventeen or eighteen, I didn't feel like I was in a minority. And it wasn't as if there hadn't been some fooling around, I told myself. There was inept fumbling on the dance floor of a school disco—literally, since we were in the corner, half buried by other people's coats, their pockets giving up their secrets each time one of us moved to wake a sleeping limb or plunge into the kiss from another angle, as if that might have helped. In a tiny Left Bank bar, I learned French kissing from a native, now remembered only as the scent of leather, the taste of Marlboro Lights, and the blush that scalded his cheeks when he afterward tried to add Metro fare dodging to

my repertoire and got us both caught. *"Je suis anglaise,"* I told the
uniformed official, who had whipped out a notebook and was
threatening a fat fine. It was the second time that evening that I'd
invoked my nationality as an excuse for not knowing how things
were done.

At university, I fell asleep beside a pale boy who claimed that his
room once belonged to E. M. Forster and then passed out. In the middle of another night in another room, another boy leaped out of bed
to take a cold shower. With a third boy, it was I who leaped out of bed,
though I headed not to the shower block but back to my own room.

While I didn't have a sense of being choosy, exactly—there were
too few opportunities to feel that way—I suppose I was waiting. I
knew there was only one first time and didn't want to be burdened
with a memory I'd spend my whole life trying to forget. I also sensed
how badly it could go, having watched other girls get dropped by
boys the moment they went to bed with them. Plus, there was the
fact that the longer I waited, the more careful I had to be about de-
ciding: if it was getting to seem freakish to me that I was still a virgin,
the wrong boy might easily be unnerved. And then there was this:
what if I was simply no good at it? Though welcome week had
brought a deluge of handy pamphlets to supplement peer-group lore
and agony-aunt advice pages (they were intended to promote safe
sex but had plenty about sex in general), there was no getting over
the fact that I was unpracticed. My grandmother's generation had
worried about getting pregnant; mine worried about technique.

It's been many decades since virginity was something prized in
secular society, and, having left behind my teenage years, I was
beginning to sense that my own was something to get rid of, quickly.
Given another six months or so, I might have considered throwing
myself at the next willing male, simply to get it over with. Except

that the other thing I craved was devotion intense enough to anes-
thetize me against any embarrassment or physical pain that the
event might entail. If only I could find a boy I adored enough, I
could deal with him realizing that it was my first time, discovering
my lack of finesse. Then along came Dan.

That first time was worth the wait. It was also dramatic—melo-
dramatic, you could say—and neither of these facts has stood me in
particularly good stead in the years since. Here is how it happened.
We'd been to a barbecue together. Though I'd grown up in Norfolk,
my mother and younger sister had moved to London when I started
university, and so the family home was now a rundown garden flat
whose oddly shaped rooms ran off a long, leafy corridor. The barbecue
was a few minutes' drive away in a big curvy bowl of a park, ringed
by what appeared to be a picket fence but was in fact molded concrete.
It took us a few laps to find a parking space, and rather than walk
back round to the gate, we decided to clamber right over. It wasn't
high, but just being beside Dan made me feel dizzy. Swinging my
legs over and leaping down, I snagged my skirt and slipped, my knee
scraping the fence as the fabric slowly tore. I was mortified. I was
also hurting, but the mortification trumped the pain. The blood
disturbed Dan, who drove me directly home. No one else was in,
and I quickly dabbed at my cuts, covering them with Band-Aids and
jeans. My ruined skirt I left abandoned in a tattered, bloody heap
on the bathroom floor.

We went back to the barbecue and drank punch from plastic
beakers. The afternoon wore on, and at some point, with evening
nearing, we extricated ourselves, leaving the car behind and taking
the train to Dan's. He lived in the suburbs, far enough out for the
underground to become overground, flashing past shopping centers
and tower blocks strung with laundry while the sky blazed pink

with summer promise. Later, on the floor of his boyhood bedroom, I lost the virginity that had lately begun to feel a burden.

"I'm starting to fall in love with you," Dan told me as we sat tangled up in each other. Outside, the light had mellowed and weekend sounds drifted up to us: a car crunching up a drive, doors slamming and children squabbling. Inside, it was different. His father had died just eighteen months previously, and the house had an abandoned feel to it. Downstairs, rooms seemed shut up even with his sister sprawled on the telephone and the television lighting up dark corners. It had been built in the thirties on a cul-de-sac lined with identical homes, detached and optimistic by design, but whenever we arrived there at the end of an evening, it would look somehow grainier than its neighbors, set farther back from the curb, crouching like a toad behind its knotted front garden. Love in that house—even student love, hungry and headlong—felt like a life raft.

Did I stay over that night? I don't remember, but sooner or later I arrived back home to find my mother furious with worry. Though she knew where I'd gone, at some point in the evening it occurred to her that I still hadn't returned. It was probably about then that she spotted the heap of fabric in the bathroom. She'd helped me pick out that skirt the day before and knew how pleased I'd been with it. Now it lay on the floor, rent and bloodstained. In hindsight, it was almost Grecian—comically so—but my mother happens to be a big fan of crime dramas, and as she stood in the bathroom clutching that bloodied rag, it must have seemed more like *NYPD Blue*.

Ever since, I've expected sex to come with drama and love. I've usually managed to create the drama, but the love has been harder to come by. It didn't last with Dan. During the months after graduation—the summer months, which we were still too institutionalized to view as anything other than free time—we trod water.

Beneath the calm surface, we were all a bit frantic. Either we'd accepted jobs and were preparing for the beginning of the end, as we saw it, or else we were stupefied by possibility. It seemed that each stage of our education had prepared us for only more education, leaving us with no hint of what we were supposed to do now. Those with funds headed off to bury their heads in faraway sands. The rest of us temped and wondered what to do next. Dan and I had planned to save up and go to France for a month or so, but as July became August, we couldn't seem to make any progress.

One night we sat in my mother's garden, surrounded by the debris of dinner while waxy candle stubs guttered into darkness. It was just the two of us, out there with the moths, as life—real life, with alarm clocks and pension plans—stilled in the surrounding houses. Autumn hovered in the sighing trees, but it was balmy enough, and here and there windows hung open, each containing a little lit stage—a tableau of how a person might choose to live, of what we were supposed to want. In the summer-scented night, buzzed with rosé, I sensed what had been so close almost a year earlier on the shore of Lake Kinneret: the exhilarating blankness of my own future. It had felt too big to seize back then, but now I was ready for it. Well, I had to be, because here it was. Did I try to explain this to Dan, or did I merely glance over to see if he felt it, too? When he accepted a place in a law conversion course a few weeks later, it seemed he was choosing more than just another year of certainty. The morning that I knew I had to end it, I realized what *just* sex was. That last time, it seemed like cheating on who we'd been.

By then, I'd started working in publishing. It wasn't exactly the job I wanted—I was still figuring out what that might be—but it came with a desk and a title, and there were doughnuts on Fridays. It had drama, too, because the imprint's main title was *The Guinness*

Book of World Records, and my days were spent dealing with extremes of scale and ambition—the largest, the loudest, the most every-thingest. Even as I lived it, that first autumn in the adult world felt as vivid as memory: bright and breezy and so warm that I strolled bare-legged into October and a future that at last seemed mine to inscribe, thrilled through and through. If Dan had felt something of that, we probably would have lasted a little longer, though I don't kid myself that we wouldn't have outgrown each other sooner rather than later. Besides, I'd fallen for another—my heart now belonged to boundless, inconstant possibility. Had I been seduced by the fickle idea that someone more perfect might be waiting around the corner? I had, but it wasn't only that—I also believed a more perfect me could be waiting there, too, just beyond the turn in the road.

That restlessness sent me skittering into a career in literary jour-nalism, pulling together a life of deadlines and parties and an un-healthy diet of fiction. In one year alone, I reviewed more than two hundred novels. Slender tomes by big names, featherweight door-stops, whodunits and thrillers—almost all contained a love story. I charged through my twenties with the haphazard velocity of a champagne cork. I danced in restaurants, flirted in Soho clubs and argued about books in after-hours drinking dives. I wasn't earning much, but as every rookie hack learns, the free social life provided by junkets and press launches can nicely fatten a lean starter salary. If you consumed enough canapés you could convince yourself you'd had dinner, and by the time the fizz ran out you wouldn't be able to taste the next morning's headache in the plonk that replaced it. I was young and living in London, renting a tiny studio flat with a kitchenette and a sofa bed and, when the trees lost their leaves, an intoxicating view of the city's skyline.

They were fun, giddy times, and if ever anyone had taken me

aside and questioned whether I wasn't having too much fun, I would have smiled away their doubts. I was just making up for a nonexistent adolescence marooned in the middle of Norfolk. Wasn't this why I'd worked so hard, to escape to the bright lights and the big city? And I was still working hard, writing through the night at least once a week and often through the weekends, too. I skipped holidays and blew any spare cash I had on black cabs, which quickly became an addiction. There is something uniquely extravagant about their roomy interiors and glossy exteriors. I'd first fallen for them on a childhood trip up to town. Torrential rain had flooded streets in northwest London, and when my favorite great-uncle collected us from the station it was in his cab, which wasn't actually black but burgundy. While other vehicles gave up, we sailed on through. He wasn't the only cabbie in the family, and this knowledge somehow made handing over the extortionate fare a humbling experience. During the hectic years that followed graduation, cabs became nothing less than a kind of mobile confessional for me. Their glassed-off interiors enforced rare moments of quiet and solitude, and if the driver was chatty, the anonymity inspired unexpected truths as the night-filled streets scrolled by. It was while sitting alone on those vast, slippery seats that I would occasionally let myself wonder where all this ambition-fueled fun was going.

On some deep-down level, I think I regarded my singleness as part of the deal. I told myself I was looking for something more meaningful, more lasting, yet I consistently chose entanglements with men who weren't really available or keen enough to commit, men who were emotionally or geographically unreachable. Often, even their years made them remote to me. What they had in common was that they were unlikely to impinge too much on a life that seemed to be the one I wanted. By comparison with the relationships

I witnessed around me—couples bickering in the tinned-goods aisle at the supermarket, the love that seemed more like an insecure habit clung on to from university—there was even a certain mascara-smudged glamour to the unpredictability of it all. And if nothing else, these liaisons made for some good stories.

There was the boy who showed me the way out on the way into his apartment, explaining how the locks worked in case I should want to flee while he was sleeping. (The block had a talking elevator, and I couldn't help noticing how depressed the recorded woman's voice sounded as she counted us up floor by floor.) One man carried me to his bed then bid me lick his face (while looking him in the eye), and another wanted me to wear a burka he'd brought back from Afghanistan (I refused—it seemed offensive on every level). There was the engaged novelist (I didn't know it), the much older, almost divorced novelist (I didn't believe it), and the aspiring novelist, who promised me that he was such a good lover, I'd kick myself forever afterward if I said no (I said no).

Sure enough, each successive liaison went the way of the one before, either before it had gotten started or after a torrid few months. Left feeling foolish, I'd do what comes so naturally to women and mock myself. Often, my audience was The Group. We were all at university together, but in the years since, we've drifted in an improbable array of directions. Flora teaches up north while Becky is in children's telly in London. Priya is flying high in finance and Lucy makes documentaries. Sara, a solicitor, has been married for three years already, and Neil, an honorary member since the rest of us all attended the same Oxbridge college—a girls-only school—may as well be married, having been with the same boyfriend far longer than anyone but Sara.

We get together less than we used to as a group, but that's still how we think of ourselves, and it's against The Group's achievements that we continue to measure our own, even where romance is concerned. We'd be catching up on one another's office flirtations or old flames when Flora would turn to me. "Come on, you've always got some guy on the go." And so I'd fill them in, trying not to notice how sometimes the humor backfired and I'd see sympathy or, worse still, pity in their eyes as they listened to me ham up the hopelessness of it all. Tellingly, I cast the men—even the much older novelist—as boys and myself as a girl. Yes, while it mostly was fun, part of me knew that this wasn't just fooling around, and that even if I didn't sleep with each of those men, it was all somehow taking its toll, if only in the way others perceived me. Another question was niggling in the back of my mind, too: at what point does *popular* become a euphemism for a clutch of less desirable traits?

After one of my midtwenties birthday parties, a friend asked me for another's number, adding that he wasn't sure if she was single. "She had that girlfriend look," he said, sighing. What was that look, I wondered, and when did I lose it? I began to make a list in my head of the men I had slept with, wondering whether my tally was disproportionate, wondering why I cared so much. Weren't we supposed to be free of all that? I started to feel spooked by news stories of rising cases of STIs and STDs. I'd have heart-to-hearts with a friend of my mum's who'd say, "You don't want to end up like me," which was heartbreaking to hear: she was so accomplished and well liked that the singleness and childlessness she was cautioning against seemed but minor details, yet for her they appeared defining.

We had come of age in muddled times, my girlfriends and I. Raised to believe we could do anything the boys could—that we could even do wrong like Margaret Thatcher, who was in power for most of our childhoods—we felt uneasy leaving our coed comprehensives for an all-women's college a lot like the one she'd attended after grammar school.

In our world, there was no need for such a place. We had no interest in feminism, either, which seemed to have argued itself into irrelevance decades earlier. We'd reaped the benefits and moved on. When the going got tough, we turned up the volume on our radios and reminded ourselves that "Girls Just Want to Have Fun"—an eighties song, I know, but we were precociously nostalgic, and besides, the alternative was Girl Power, whatever that meant.

Teaching just across town was Germaine Greer, and if ever we'd thought to pick up a copy of the book that made her name, we might have been surprised. *The Female Eunuch* turned twenty-one the year before I reached the age of consent (and the year after one of my fifteen-year-old classmates became a mother, following in the footsteps of her sister, who had given birth in the school loos). In a foreword to the anniversary edition, Professor Greer had this to say: "Twenty years ago it was important to stress the right to sexual expression and far less important to underline a woman's right to reject male advances; now it is even more important to stress the right to reject penetration by the male member, the right to safe sex, the right to chastity, the right to defer physical intimacy until there is irrefutable evidence of commitment." We didn't seek out this wisdom, however, and had it been lit up before us on a lecture-hall projector, we'd have thought that the "woman" she spoke of was someone else, not us. We were postfeminist. Weren't we?

We graduated into the era of the ladette. Boozy, brawling and out of control, the ladette was at least honest about who she was: one of the boys. And that, it seemed, was the net victory of all those burned bras—they had won us the right to behave exactly like men.

Or as men were perceived to behave, because it wasn't clear that they had much more of an idea of their role in life than we did. Still, when it came to relationships, I followed the boys' lead. Neediness was the biggest crime, and so I got angry and sad on my own. We may have been sexually empowered, but we were also emotionally frustrated.

Technology seemed only to underscore our disempowerment. As if sitting by the phone weren't bad enough, we now had to take the phone with us and hear its silence in cafés and bars. As one male "dating pro" bragged in an article by marriage expert and Manhattan Institute fellow Kay S. Hymowitz, text messages "deflect from unnecessary personal involvement and keep women on edge." Courtship, if that's what it was, stepped up its pace—texting didn't only deflect, it encouraged us to abbreviate, just as e-mailing had us dropping formalities like capital letters. As we cut to the chase, it wasn't only the rules of grammar that were being compromised.

One time in my early twenties, I dented a wall by hurling my phone at it rather than risking a needy-seeming text. On buses, I'd hear other women, mostly around my age, grumbling into their own phones about unreadable silences and baffling behavior. They were angry—in their own way, just as angry as those repressed suburban housewives who inspired Betty Friedan's *The Feminine Mystique*, another book that, if asked about, I'd have said we'd moved far, far beyond.

Somewhere along the way, the speed date had been born, but it was quickly surpassed by online dating. Why waste precious minutes on face-to-face interaction when you could scroll through potential mates preselected by a computer? Eyes were no longer meeting across crowded rooms; people were shopping online for a cute smile and compatible music collections. Soon, *connecting* was redefined as something that required the click of a mouse rather than that other click—the mysterious, indefinable kind without which a relationship is doomed, no matter how perfectly matched two people seem on one another's laptop screens. It all brought us closer together yet kept us apart.

Back when I broke up with Dan, I had thought my curiosity would be fulfilled by another Dan—a slightly older one, perhaps, one who'd already become the person I'd wanted mine to be, who lived in the world I hoped to make my own. That was not how it turned out. If anything connected my twentysomething dating experiences, it was a profound disconnectedness. Unfortunately, the moment I fell into bed with a man, I'd fall at least a little in love. Was it biological? Was I responding to the notionally dead double standard—a double standard lively enough for women to continue scaling down their sexual conquests while men fibbed upward? And was it really so unreasonable of me to stubbornly link sex and love?

Whatever the reason, through all that fun threaded a trail of crumpled, tear-soggy tissues—the kind that confetti your laundry when left, forgotten, in a pocket. Even as I sobbed through my breakup with Dan, a lurking suspicion told me that time would ease the hurt, that it would bring more and ease more, and that it would all toughen me up. One washed-out July, a few months before that New York serendipity, I sat in a cooling bathtub reflecting on how my latest lover had slipped off the radar. I'd grown so tough that I didn't care enough to cry—a realization that immediately brought hot tears plopping into the sudsy water. At the time, the gaggle of fictional heroines we were offered was led by the likes of Bridget Jones and Carrie Bradshaw—funny women never more engaging than when they were feeling blue or getting into clownish scrapes—but this was becoming tedious.

Back in London, my sparkly ring is on my desk when a chance e-mail exchange with a forgotten mutual friend reveals that in all likelihood, Dan and I really had passed shoulder-to-shoulder on Fifth Avenue. He'd apparently flown out to New York with his girlfriend that same week and she had traveled home his fiancée, perhaps even tilting her hand to admire a De Beers dazzler somewhere high above the Atlantic.

Sometimes, it seems as if life's biggest lessons teach us only what we already know: the heartbreak that makes true the catchy pop refrain; the misstep that illustrates the nursery fable; or, for me, the coincidence that proved fact to be far, far stranger than any amount of fiction. To have ended up in that same city, on that same street, at the exact same moment—it was as if some cosmic joker had gathered up the fabric of my twenties and given it a good shake. It was so fabulously unlikely that it felt like a gift—maybe even a bit of New York magic—a feat of such uncanny synchronicity that it had to mean something. But what?

Manhattan has grown to represent all the restless, striving momentum of those years, so it's ironic that it was there that I should have been forced to pause, to stand still even as the city's bright clamor washed over me, and to hazard a glance back. Replaying it in my head as I watch the falling glitter reveal the emptiness of my five-dollar ring, I can no longer resist another fact: Dan had been my first, and after almost a decade of dead-ended seconds, thirds, fourths and, yes, more—he was also the last to have told me "I love you." I didn't need a ring; I needed only to hear those words.

TWO

... *And My Last*

Give me chastity and continency—but not yet!

—St. Augustine, *Confessions*

A few weeks after that chance e-mail revealed the extent of my Manhattan coincidence, I find myself sharing the story on a first date. Across the table from me sits Jake, a man I met some years earlier at a dinner to celebrate a novel—a romance, as it happens. It was held in a higgledy-piggledy town house with perilous stairs and low ceilings, hidden amid the mazelike streets that seam London's heart—the kind of place that appears to have dropped out of time, giving the dangerous impression that nothing that occurs within its sloping four walls counts out in the world beyond. While everyone milled around, drinking too quickly on empty stomachs, we struck up a conversation, and when we found we'd been seated beside each other, we carried on.

Ours was a small table so there was a lot of group chat, but we two ended each conversation between ourselves. I don't think we talked about anything momentous—what we each did (he is a trans-lator), whom we knew and how, the usual. He was a little on the short side, had around a decade on me and wore sneakers. Already a critic by then, I didn't check off the good points—his breath-catching smile, his quick, dark gaze, the bodily pull of his charm—but I felt them. Though the dinner ran late, Jake left early. Saying his good-byes, he paused to squeeze my shoulder before turning to leave. As I watched him, an odd thought popped into my head: He'll do.

These words may not sound like the stuff of latent infatuation, but for me they have extra resonance. My favorite great-aunt, a woman of elegantly bluff wisdom, has been married to my favorite great-uncle—the cabbie—for more than sixty years. Go round for tea, and he will still ask you to move your chair if it's obstructing his view of her. Their account of their courtship is a wonderful tale of pursuit that might today be seen as stalking. It ducks and dives down a series of alleyways, but it begins when he glimpsed her in the cinema. When the credits rolled, he followed her home on the bus. Luckily for him, London's East End was still a small enough place that my grandfather, the eldest of her several brothers, knew exactly who he was, and knew, too, that he was as all right as any man would ever be to woo his little sister.

My great-uncle remains dapper and my great-aunt queenly, still the dreamy only granddaughter my great-great-grandfather would sit on a cushion in the window of his upholstery workshop, a prin-cess to show off to his passing friends. But as that well-told tale un-folds, they become who they were back then: a young man made plucky by passion, and a shy girl who knew exactly what she was do-ing. What makes it comical is the bit where my great-aunt adds: "I said to myself, he'll do." There it is, this sweet love story, under-pinned by pragmatism. She is a very particular person in every detail of her life, so there is nothing offhand about her assessment. She meant he would do to spend the rest of her life with—and really, when it comes to that, how certain can any of us ever be? To this day, I've only ever thought that of one man: Jake. I couldn't have guessed his real role in my story—that he would ultimately set me on the path to chastity.

After that dinner, I dreamed up some tenuous work premise to e-mail him, though he didn't reply. He had a girlfriend, of course. Now I'd know it immediately, but even then I suspected as much. A couple of years passed, and occasionally, having darted down yet another romantic rabbit hole, I'd think of him, the one who'd do, slip-sliding away into the night.

When we next ran into each other at a party, he had to be reintroduced to me before I recognized him. "You e-mailed me," he said, with a playful hint of smugness. I must have liked him quite a bit, I reflected, wondering whether unresolved attraction had an expiry date, or whether we don't always remain loyal to its initial tug in some small way. But I'd had enough of that party, and besides, over in the corner stood my most recent dalliance, a man who'd apparently lost his phone and been locked out of both his e-mail accounts—for a whole ten days—then tried to get me to go on holiday with him and his six-year-old daughter. ("He wants you to play nanny!" was honorary Group-member Neil's outraged response.) And did I mention that the party was to toast a book about pickup artists? It was time to leave.

Cut to another gathering, maybe six months on. It's a Monday evening, and the room is filled with publishers from abroad, adrift in their foreign week and keen to rock on, drinking and dancing into the small hours like middle-aged men at a work conference— which they largely are. Allure is a quicksilver thing. Too ephemeral to be studied, it brushes all of us from time to time. You can't see it yourself, but you can sometimes feel it in the wry smile of an ex or the sly gaze that trails you down a street. It was happening to me that evening—one of those perfect moments when everything that you know to be fleeting seems briefly bright enough to believe in. I'd gone along half hoping to find another person altogether—a harmless flirtation that I knew would come to nothing—and it was that other person's face that I scanned the crowd for when I arrived. He wasn't there, but I spotted my friend Caroline instead, and nudging my way through the heaving shoulders of the dancing throng, I didn't see that the man she was talking to was Jake until I'd reached her side and he'd turned that smile on me. This time, I recognized him.

Together we made ourselves a corner in the melee and huddled close to be heard, our breathy words whispered—well, yelled—into each other's ears. By the time the lights came up and the bouncers signaled that the party was over, it was almost three in the morning. I went to get my coat and came back to find him looking for me. He drove me home through streets that were eerily deserted. Cruising across an overpass high above empty, glowing offices, we had three lanes to ourselves. The traffic lights switched from red to green only for us. It was as if we'd crossed over into dreamtime.

When I kissed him good night, first on one cheek and then on the other, I hesitated for a beat, our eyes meeting just long enough for me to feel my own close, and then his lips on mine, impossibly tender. There was something else, too: he preempted my every move. As I lifted my hand to touch his cheek, his fingers touched mine. As I thought about kissing his eyelids, there were his lips brushing mine. It was as if I'd found a twin. He slipped his hands from the lapels of my coat to the V of skin left bare by my dress. "I can feel your heart," he told me, his eyes gleaming in the dark, liquid and alive. In the thrill of that moment, I felt like he was claiming it, and for a split second was ready to surrender everything to him, just like that.

He still had a girlfriend, of course—the same German photographer who'd been on the scene ever since we first met. Does it make it any less treacherous that she was now in Mexico indefinitely, that she had been gone for months already? Following him to his car that night, kissing on the sleeping street, I'd felt sassy and in control. Pulling back to look at him, this figure from my unrealized past, I decided he'd been sent as Cupid's envoy, a reminder that sometimes things work out. *Don't give up hope* seemed to be the meaning of it all—*hang on in there.* It wasn't about Jake; he was just the messenger. And yes, he had a girlfriend. Yet even in that moment, when I was fully prepared to step out of his steamed-up car and close the door quietly on all our breathless wonderment, I couldn't help offering up a little knock-on-wood prayer that maybe this mightn't be so theoretical after all. What if it were straightforwardly about him, me, him-and-me?

It was folly and I knew it. His relationship seemed to be over, but the fact that he was clinging to it only made it clearer that he was in no position to become involved with another. Still, when he asked for my number, I gave it. "Call me," I said, cooler than I've ever managed before or since. I smiled as I let myself in. I smiled as I swept off the evening's makeup and felt the tenderness in my lips, as I set my alarm for just a few hours' time. Drifting toward sleep, I was still smiling when he texted me a good-night.

In the days that followed, I replayed our kisses and caresses, certain that they were enough. Nevertheless, each time I answered a text, another would appear, and each time another appeared, I'd answer. In the bleeping to and fro of our messages, tantalizing expectations resonated; we were daring each other to meet. At the same time, my anxiety was mounting. When dinner was finally suggested, I purposely set the date for a week later, giving us seven days to realize what a bad idea it was. We didn't—or if we did, we ignored it. Suddenly, there we were: date night.

The restaurant was subterranean and Spanish, too big and impersonal-feeling for its menu's rustic notes. The first to arrive, I stood at the bar trying to regain some of that poise I'd felt ten days previously. By the time he edged in, bringing the cold from outside on his jacket and blustering apologies for lateness, I'd added a precarious cocktail to my awkwardness.

In some ways, it was a dreadful first date. Too full of butterflies to eat, we opted for a tapas menu whose dishes were small but so numerous we had to annex the next-door table. Eventually, our talking ground to a halt along with our eating. What remained was meltingly intense eye contact. It was so potent it felt unseemly, and I glanced round, flushed, half expecting to meet the stares of other diners. Finding a path through the untouched plates, he took my hand.

Afterward, we made our way back to his office. He had to collect something and then he'd drive me home, he said, though we both knew this was only partly true. We were already entangled as we covered those few wintry streets. There was snow on the air and the wind whipped our cheeks while he danced a cold jig, patting his pockets for keys. Hauling open a large warehouse door, he gestured through a dismal hallway and out into a courtyard, where a fire escape rose like a beanstalk. Higher and higher we climbed, my heels ringing out on the metal steps as we ascended to that urban altitude where offices give way to roof terraces and straggly sunflowers, skeletal reminders of warmer times. Inside, it smelled of paraffin heaters. He spun me round, kissing me in profile, leaning to the left a little, then to the right, as if trying to peer around my edges, to see where I ended. "You're too much," he told me. I smiled at his adoration—so serious, so unexpected—and he eyed my neck, shiveringly vampiric, tracing its contour with his tongue, while from the window beyond, the phosphorescent night made silhouettes of us. He was too, too much.

That was how we began. I'd turned thirty by then, and though I'd seen Dan ring-shopping in New York just a few months before, I still hadn't quite figured out what to make of it. With the moment's significance hovering close, I knew only that I had to make this new relationship mean something—it had to add up to something in a way that none of my twentysomething flings and hookups and aimless dalliances ever had. I wasn't going to sleep with him, of course, not until he'd resolved the situation with his absentee girlfriend.

He didn't. I did.

I'd like to gloss over this failure of resolve, but the circumstances are significant, because my decision wasn't determined by a sense of his ardor ebbing but my own. Earlier on, we'd been sitting in a pub when I became aware of him sniping at things around us: a girl's chubby back exposed by her low-rise jeans, the gaucheness of a grown-up family perusing bar menus. Silly stuff, but mean-sounding. Until that moment, our connection had felt so essential that minor— even major—differences in lifestyle, opinion, and age had seemed to burn up in our orbit. When I sensed them starting to slip through, I gave in to sex as a way of obscuring them.

For a while, it worked. There were early-hours assignations, breathless texts, kisses so epic they left us both stunned. Youthful excess had imposed sobriety on Jake, and since he was teetotal, I rarely drank when we were together, yet I felt light-headed just looking at him. The sex blotted out everything, including the fact that I was sleeping with another woman's boyfriend. It even obscured the true meaning of the words that accompanied each rueful parting. Yet if I'd listened carefully—really carefully—to those words rather than to my feelings, I would have known that he still hadn't made any definite steps toward formalizing the breakup with his girl-friend; that he didn't even have a time frame in mind. I would have known that when he said he didn't want to mislead me with prom-ises, he really wasn't making any. I would also have known that whatever he said, I'd go ahead and mislead myself anyhow, glossing it with all that I was aching to hear. Or perhaps that was the one thing I did know.

Eventually, I couldn't hold out any longer. I started listening, and this was what I heard: "I'm not in love with you." He said it in those exact words and in such a way that I felt a fool for ever having thought that he might have been. The voice that I knew thick with early-morning passion or scratchy with late-night longing was sud-denly steady and matter-of-fact, not even warmed by protest. Truth can be as exhilarating as sex itself, an exchange of confidences as intimate as waking together at first light. Initially I felt numbed. Then incredulous. How could he have experienced a fraction of what I had when we were together and deny that there was some-thing deeper between us? Was I experiencing that alone? And if not, could he really believe that something so powerful was *just* sex? Or was I merely confusing lust with love?

It was the tentative beginning of spring, and as that fickle season advanced, hopelessness rolled in like squally showers. This much was abundantly clear: I'd once again gone to bed with someone who wasn't in love with me. I had dearly wanted this relationship to be momentous, and in a way, it was. While no man since Dan had said that he loved me, none had explicitly told me what Jake did, that he *didn't* love me.

It all came to a head outside my favorite bar. It is hidden inside a Mayfair hotel that has always struck me as so enchanted I've been known to swing through its revolving doors simply to breathe in the lobby's fragrant air before spinning back out into the real world. That magic does not extend to the pavement outside, it transpires.

I was shortly heading off to New York again—to be a bridesmaid, ironically—but before that, Jake had to go to Barcelona. On my return, we would miss each other by hours at Heathrow as he headed out to Mexico—yes, for a wedding also, and yes, with his estranged girlfriend. Faced with a three-week separation and the knowledge that she would be at his side, my version of our story—the version in which he really would finish with her, the version that I'd sustained as an act of will—finally revealed itself as the fantasy it had always been. This was a kind of good-bye, I realized, a farewell to fictive love.

There were tears; of course there were tears. Startled by my crying—it wasn't the pretty kind—Jake became solicitous, putting me in a taxi and promising to drive round and check up on me after his business dinner. He kept his promise, even though he first reversed into a Dumpster and smashed his rear window, which he then had to tape up. It was three o'clock in the morning by the time he arrived on my doorstep, and the birds were singing as he headed off again. He called from the airport and again midway through my week in New York.

Yet after all that, he didn't exit so much as drift from my life. We both returned to London and for two months I heard nothing from him. I stubbornly refused to call him—he'd said he would call me, but I also knew that I'd done all I could. The silence was at last growing bearable when he rang. Seeing his name, I dropped my phone and let voice mail pick up. I wasn't quite shaking but I did feel physi-

cally shaken. The next day I returned his call—I couldn't resist—
and when he suggested we meet up, I couldn't resist that, either.

The city was melting in a heat wave. Its pubs had taken on the
look of mirages and the wooded corners of the nearby park were
crammed with picnickers, sun-flushed and slow, ringed by wilting
children and tubs of limp salad. Balls sailed through the air trailed
by the eyes of soccer players and dogs too hot to give chase, until
they too plunked to the ground and trickled to a halt, giving in to a
contagious torpor. Every item of clothing I owned felt too hot, too
heavy, so it wasn't really surprising that we ended up back at Jake's,
naked.

I didn't know it at the time, but that molten July night when it
was too hot to think from one heartbeat to the next would be etched
in my mind over the coming months. I would wish that I'd paused
to record each lip print, each gentle caress of rough thumb, to remember the way that our kisses grew so greedy our teeth clashed—
deliciously—or how our bodies twinned so well together from our
faces all the way down to our toes. Even our breath seemed to fit. If
I'd known then what I was about to sign up for, I might have found
a way to preserve just a drop of the experience's essence.

Later on that night, the rain came—a gentle hiss that intensified
through the early hours as we finally slept, lulled by its insistence. I
woke, too early to feel rested, into a day that was already muggy
and close, as if the rainfall had been but a dream. Rather than promise relief, the gray sky lidded the humidity and turned dawn's sounds
tinny—a cat's howl, a mewling baby, the first siren. Somewhere up
above, a red-eye rumbled like thunder. My own dry spell had barely
begun.

.   .   .

In the immediate aftermath of that sizzling interlude, I vainly hoped that it might prove to be a beginning rather than the real end. I gazed back shiftily whenever I caught my own eye in the mirror. Over the next couple of weeks, Jake and I texted and chatted but we did not see each other. On the morning of his birthday he revealed that he was in America. He texted me his return date, too, which somehow made it worse—as if I'd want to pick up my forlorn pursuit as soon as he was back. I'd had no idea that he was planning a trip, and even though he claimed to be on the opposite side of the border to his girlfriend, the gaping geographical distance meant I could no longer resist the emotional distance that he'd been insisting on throughout. Verbally, at least, he had been honest. I'd deluded myself better than any lover could. I'd let my body tell me that it was being made love to—real love.

Looking back, I saw that this was a recurring problem of mine. Jake was an extreme example, but the pattern was there: as soon as I went to bed with a man, I'd lose any clear sense of perspective. I had consistently mistaken casual hookups for rose-tinted beginnings.

However uninvolved I started out—however uninvolved it seemed I was supposed to be—I could not remain cool-headed (or -hearted) as the temperature shot up.

To admit as much felt like letting down the sisterhood. I knew that as a woman, my right to sexual expression was hard won, yet that ideal seemed to have been watered down to become intimacy without intimacy. While it is billed as empowering to be able to love and leave a man like a man, to me it felt like I was denying a whole set of instinctive feminine responses, forcing myself to conform to decidedly masculine relationship ideals. And what a waste of energy all this weeping seemed!

In Jake's case, the existence of an absentee girlfriend made it screamingly clear that I should not have slept with him, but what of the guys who preceded him? My mother, an increasingly reluctant if still sympathetic listener to my tales of romantic woe, had honed her response to a single-note lament: "You sleep with these men too soon." An artist who came of age in the sixties and met my father in a hippie commune, she is no prude. Her refrain sounded deeply unfashionable, yet I couldn't help thinking: might she be right? It's true that there seemed to be a fundamental disconnect between my thoughts on sex and romance, between what I desired and what I yearned for. I'd had enough sex without love; maybe it was time to look for love without sex?

There seemed just one way to test it: a year of chastity. It was a drastic response, but in the weepy aftermath of one more failed liaison, that was what made it so appealing. The more I thought about it, the more interesting and alarming the proposition seemed. Might it change the kind of men I attracted and my response to them? After all, walking away had been an option in every instance. Would it enable me to fall back in love with romance, rather than eyeing it mistrustfully as the prelude to yet another tear-streaked denouement? Would I actually be able to last twelve months?

And then I stopped myself. Did I really want to do this? Let's face it, we all know what dry spells feel like. Though there's no exact definition of how long you need to go before you're officially in one, you sure as anything know it when you're there. It begins with a feeling of invisibility—a foggy fading around the edges. Next, it seems that instead of inhabiting your body, you're hibernating within it. It doesn't entirely feel like your body, either—its contours are more memory than reality. Eventually, it's as if a glass wall were separating you from everyone else on this planet, because everyone but you is having sex. Soon, every ad that appears on the telly, every magazine cover story, every chart-topping single piped out in the supermarket—all of this feels aimed at them, the people who are having all the sex that you're not having.

For Voltaire, chastity was a vice; for Aldous Huxley, a perversion. "We may eventually come to realize that chastity is no more a virtue than malnutrition," declared Alex Comfort, whose famed manual introduced bondage and swinging to Middle America (while devoting just four sentences to the clitoris).

Malnutrition? Was that what I was signing up for?

As I sat wondering whether or not I had the stamina for such a bizarre-seeming experiment, a conversation drifted back to me from a few months before. My friend Freddie is a joker with a disarmingly earnest streak, a dedicated partygoer (his enviably thick business cards describe him as an events executive) who likes retro suits and sharp shoes. We'd arranged to catch up over drinks in a slick new bar he wanted to try out. The cocktail list was the length of a novella, and I was still paging through it when he announced that he was in love. I looked up cautiously. Freddie had fallen in love before and his feelings tended not to be reciprocated, so my heart clenched in anticipation of what might be in store for him.

He'd liked the girl in question for years, he began—so far, so familiar. They were friends, and despite his devotion, she seemed happy to leave it at that. It was as friends that they'd met for dinner—one of those perfect, chatty meals that stretch beyond dessert, beyond coffee, all the way to a shared final glass. As the restaurant emptied around them, he leaned back and gazed at her. He was completely happy, it occurred to him—happy enough to say exactly what he felt without minding how it came out. Smiling, he told her, "You know, I don't care if I never get to sleep with you."

Those words were about to prove his open sesame. He went home with her that night and they've been inseparable ever since. If it were anyone but Freddie, I'd have thought he'd used them as a shrewd chat-up line, but I knew he'd spoken with complete sincerity—she must have known it, too, because I don't think they'd have worked otherwise. It was that kind of romance I'd lost sight of, I realized. And just like that, my mind was made up.

I could never have guessed what the next twelve months would hold.

THREE

September OR *Dressing Around*

A dress should be tight enough
to show you're a woman and loose
enough to prove you're a lady.

—Edith Head, *The Dress Doctor*

The woman standing before me has more than a touch of the eighties about her. It's there in the shoulders of her jacket, so assertive they can't help but accentuate a fragility around the collarbone, where a floppy bow falls from the neck of her silk blouse. An apparition from another era, she's gone in the blink of an eyelid—an electric-blue eyelid. In her place is a well-to-do fifties housewife, the kind who spends her days waiting for cocktail hour to inject some warmth into the smile she'll greet her husband with as he returns from the office. She's curvy in Capri pants and a trim sweater, but the sixties are near and she is about to be replaced by a racier type whose shift climbs daringly up her thighs even as its tentlike shape cloaks her figure.

All these women are me, and they dance fleetingly in the mirror of a cramped dressing room as I work my way through a pile of tops and bottoms and warm winter coats. "Beware of any enterprise that requires new clothes," Thoreau cautioned, but if you let it, womanhood will demand constant wardrobe changes. Today, I am shopping for a chaste wardrobe. This is not a vintage store—I'm too squeamish about strangers' sweat for that—yet the echoes of those other epochs ring clear in this season's collections as in most. Men's fashion hasn't embraced such flighty extremes in centuries. A suit is a suit whether its trousers taper at the ankle or its jacket fastens with two buttons rather than three. It's a suit even when it isn't a suit at all, but a muted assemblage of denim and cotton twill.

I once heard two men—boys, really—chatting as they waited outside their girlfriends' cubicles. "I'm looking forward to them being thirty-five or forty," said one to the other, squinting ahead to what must have seemed an unimaginably great age. "We'll be able to show them photos of what they're wearing now and laugh—you know, like you do with pictures of your parents." The other one laughed just thinking about it, then added, with surprising compassion for a guy spending his Saturday afternoon in a women's clothing store, "We're lucky, us blokes. You can't really go wrong with trousers and a shirt."

Ridicule is never far off in womenswear. Here is Elizabeth Stuart Phelps, whose 1873 book *What to wear?* makes Trinny and Susannah sound like mistresses of diplomacy: "The Girl of the Period, sauntering before one down Broadway, is one panorama of awful surprises from top to toe. Her clothes characterize her. She never characterizes her clothes. She is upholstered, not ornamented. She is bundled, not draped. She is puckered, not folded. She struts, she does not sweep. She has not one of the attributes of nature nor of proper art. She neither soothes the eye like a flower, nor pleases it like a picture. She wearies it like a kaleidoscope. She is a meaningless dazzle of broken effects."

Me, I could be a seventies siren or a forties femme fatale. I could look earth-mother-cozy in a big, boxy cardi—the kind my own mother wears in time-faded photos where I'm a tightly swaddled speck. Here in the dressing room, every coat hanger holds an opportunity for subtle reinvention, a sharp cutout just waiting to shape whoever brings it to life. The choice is baffling; I'm clutched by a mild panic that reminds me in turn of an odd nightmare I used to have as a child—odd because it was all about owning too many clothes.

As befitted a thatched cottage in remote north Norfolk with no central heating, my girlhood wardrobe was made up of items hand-sewn, hand-knitted and hand-me-down. Anything new and shop-bought I wore to threads, so you'd have thought that such sartorial gluttony would be the stuff of—well, dreams. Yet mine became a nightmare. I was immensely troubled by the idea of having so many clothes that I forgot about a skirt, say, or a pair of corduroys with a kicky flare at the ankle (it took a while for trends to make their way across the dank East Anglian Fens). In the dream, I'd pull open a drawer and there they would be, neatly folded, unworn, the source of a lingering melancholy that would munch into my waking hours. It was as if I'd neglected a whole other potential part of myself.

That same sense returns now as I survey the clothes that are hung, draped, heaped around the dressing room, each successive combination suggesting a new me. Outside, there is no boyfriend, but I do have my sister, waiting with mounting impatience. She is one of the few people I've told about my vow so far. It's not that I intend to keep it a secret, but I do want to give myself time to adjust to the reality of it. This is unaccustomed: I haven't exactly been coy about my personal life in the past, but already something seems different. And yes, I'm bracing myself for mockery, too.

My sister didn't mock—not quite. She is single at the moment and her reaction was part gleeful solidarity, part instinctive competitiveness. "A year? I'll beat you," she wagered. While some aspects of our relationship never change, much has. I'm three years older, and as far as she is concerned, I was the one who ended childhood for her. It was I who broke it to her that we were already halfway through the summer holidays, and I who told her all about death when one of our pet guinea pigs grew quiet and strangely light to hold. I also remember chucking a pillow across her side of our room and enrolling her in my kissing class. Now that we are notionally grown up and in our own decades (I am in my thirties, she is still in her twenties), each with our own realm (words for me, pictures for her—she is a filmmaker), our roles have reversed. I charge ahead as usual, but as I make the mistakes, it's she who learns the lessons and points them out to me. Sometimes it's as if I've acquired my own big sister.

At school, I was always the one who fitted in. I made just enough friends, kept my head down and did my homework on time. My little sister would pull up the hood of her red duffel coat and stand alone in the corner of the playground, wishing herself somewhere else. A haunted house. A Hansel and Gretel forest. Anywhere would do. Our responses to identical situations—being outsiders in an ultra-insular rural community, sent to the local school with whole wheat sandwiches in our lunchboxes and weird names stitched inside our coats—were instinctive, but they've also shaped who we've become. While she is the artist rebel, I still set out to conform. I can't resist wanting to be liked. Psychologists have a term for this sort of behavior: self-monitoring, they call it, and where love and romance are concerned, the prognosis isn't good. Self-monitors, it appears, have less stable, less satisfying relationships. Ask me about

my sister's romances, and I'll tell you that while her boyfriends may
have been fewer, they have been infinitely more devoted.

This chameleon quality also means I can step into a dressing
room with an armful of mismatched clothes and look passable in
most. But right now, with the pile of discards growing, I notice that
themes are emerging from the folds of my maybe garments. They
are generous—voluminous, even, despite some gentle tailoring
around the hips and bust. They are lined in silk but cut from tweed,
wool, heavy flannel—tough fabrics, rough fabrics, nothing flimsy or
flyaway. And while there are a couple of skirts here—one swishy,
the other straight, both falling demurely to the knee—I've mostly
picked out trousers.

In my newly chaste state, my instinct is to wrap up and hide
away, and in this I'm in sync with the seasons if not with the weather.
In the city's parks and gated garden squares, on the common that I
crossed to get here, leaves are turning. If you were to peer beyond
my restless sister and the swaddled mannequins that crowd the window, you'd spy mothers and toddlers and teenage sweethearts strolling by with bare arms and flip-flopped feet. But the afternoons are
running out of heat, the shadows growing longer. The natural world
is shutting down, readying itself for a fallow period, and I am doing
something similar.

This is a source of solace, but it isn't only the seasons that I'm
keeping step with. As I push my head through the long mohair fun-
nel of a cowl-necked pullover, emerging with my hair static and
wild, I note that I'm trying to cocoon myself, and cocooning is a
certified catwalk trend. After years of hemlines rising and waists
dropping, of tops made mostly of double-sided sticky tape and
dresses that are slashed every which way, the fashionable are
swathed in all-enveloping parkas and layered knits. Dresses may be

mini, but they are as billowy as old-fashioned maternity frocks and paired with leggings that leave plenty to the imagination.

Surveying the autumn-winter collections in the *New York Times,* veteran style maven Suzy Menkes linked the trend to the street fad for skirts worn over trousers. "This covered-up look didn't originate with designers but seems to have grown organically from how Muslim women dress and how Western women feel after a decade of visible bras and diaphanous dressing."

In the comeback of leggings, she saw more than catwalk nostalgia and the enthusiasm of a generation of fashion victims who had only ever shivered through winter in sheer pantyhose and open-toed mules. "There is a suggestion of protection," she wrote. "Where leggings in the 80s were a product of new fabric technology and the exploding club scene, now they are more serious, something to finish off an outfit and help one face a more turbulent world."

As a concept, cocooning seems right for what I'm doing. I don't want to deny my sexuality or even closet it away in mothballs. It's more about refashioning my relationship with it. It's not that I've been dashing around in bottom-grazing, cleavage-boosting numbers (nor that I'll raise an eyebrow at anyone who does), but I have come to equate sexiness with a certain degree of discomfort—the throbbing feet caused by trying to run in three-inch heels, the chilly draft that décolletage invites. It's stylishness that I yearn for—heck, who doesn't?—but while sexiness doesn't top my list of priorities, it has definitely superseded comfort when I've gone clothes shopping in the past.

"If it is a relief to take your clothes off at night, be sure that something is wrong," wrote Ellen Henrietta Richards, the first American woman to earn a degree in chemistry, in the 1870s. "Clothes should not be a burden. They should be a comfort and a protection." It was hard to find comfort in the silhouettes of the late-Victorian period, still corseted despite the much-pilloried reformative efforts of the rational dress movement, which declared that no woman should have to wear more than seven pounds of underwear.

The clothes I'm picking out will grow on me, and as my year progresses, I will come to realize that they aren't as chaste as they seem today. Sheathed within their folds, I'll discover that they speak to a more grown-up femininity: womanly rather than girlish, subtler and more personal, requiring something more complex of the wearer than a tolerance for discomfort. For now, they seem an apt uniform for a chaste challenge, unlikely to give anyone the wrong idea, myself included.

Aside from garments borrowed to sleep in—the occasional boy's T-shirt, say—the last time I let myself be seen in anything as enormous as this pullover would have been more than a dozen years ago. It's at about thirteen that my outline grows blurry in the family photo albums, fuzzed by enormous sweatshirts and a moody cast. My sister is smiling brightly but I'm invariably standing back, lured into the frame at the last minute and visibly torn between a childish delight at being needed and awkward self-awareness.

Those were the days before an image could be seen and deleted instantly, back when even the snappiest snap was attended by the mysterious process of taking out the roll of film, handing it over at the drugstore to be bagged up like evidence, and returning days later to claim a stack of glossy moments, already forgotten. Even after that wait shortened to mere hours, the process of processing was brushed with an alchemy that is no longer. Yet here I am, dressed in Pepe Jeans and a baggy Benetton sweatshirt, my eyes telling the camera that already I hate this photo, that I know I'll hate the next one, too, and the one after. I'll look fat, I'll look homely, I'll look like the pimply girl who gets left till last when it comes to picking PE teams, the person nobody wants to pair up with on activity trips. My school career was spent doing everything I could to avoid becoming that girl, but looking like her seemed almost worse.

This relentless self-criticism crept in with first bras and the monthly skipped swimming lessons. To become a woman, we girls seemed to have learned, was to be cruelly judgmental of others while taking care to reserve our tartest venom for the one in the mirror. Where did this come from? In my own case, certainly not from home. My mother gave up wearing makeup before she had me and began wearing lipstick again only after I'd begun buying my own. It seemed unlikely to have come from my father, either. Though we all lived in the same house, he was a ghostly presence, preferring to keep his own hours in his own quarters. Whenever the opportunity arose—usually in the car, in mid-row, as we hurtled around rural hairpin bends—he protested against ever having wanted kids. My sister and I would be sitting in the backseat, knowing exactly how the script went: his lack of interest was at least consistent.

By the time I turned sixteen, I was wearing men's cardigans, their sleeves rolled up into fat bracelets round my wrists, their pockets stretched down to my knees. It was the Dr. Martens era, but rather than the boots that my friends wore hand-painted with flowers, I chose the shoes, cartoonishly clunky at the ends of legs covered in tights whose bright hues only drew attention to their thickness. My skirts were floral and comically ruffled, heavily influenced by a cerise silk rah-rah skirt that my mum had run up for me years earlier on the occasion of my very first disco dance. But as I'd grown older, they had grown shorter. Abbreviated into mere pelmets, they lurked like bustles beneath those sloppy woolen cardigans, which were soon flashing Lycra tops, too.

It was conflicted, ugly-duckling attire, but bizarre as it sounds, it was also a kind of uniform, identifying me as one of a band of kids with names like Ocean and Dante—and Hephzibah. Together we formed a hippieish, goth-inflected artsy gang whose parents were predominantly Not from Round Here. There was a sporty equivalent of that same uniform—sneakers, tracksuit bottoms, boyish vests—come summer. On both sides of the senior high divide, we were getting ready to shimmy out of those cocoons, to follow where the bolder girls, the ones who'd left school just as soon as they could, had already gone. But for the time being, we were taking refuge in grungy androgyny.

While we girls were both vanishing and growing, swamped in supersized tops that made us feel tiny within while taking up a lot of space without, a portion of the boys were wearing their hair long and wriggling into skin-tight black denim that they topped with skimpy, bejeweled biker jackets. Their heavy-metal T-shirts shouted about death and destruction but their skin was still soft, their eyes clear.

One of those boys—Chris, whose hair was the darkest and glossiest—let it be known on the school grapevine that he liked me, but only after he'd lopped off those long locks and grown serious. We were going out, technically, which translated as roaming the school grounds engaged in long, serious discussions. His parents had just split up, mine were in the process of formalizing their divorce, and from this ill-omened material we tried to forge our own relationship.

I don't think we actually went out once, not alone. He'd recently passed his driving test, so there were a few intense drives home through country darkness after group pub outings, the two of us sitting side by side as his car filled with a noxious blend of hormones and timidity. We were both glad when I hopped out and wove my way toward my front door, tipsy on Strongbow. He never plucked up the nerve to move things on, and I was in a dreamy daze about ever having been picked by him.

Until then, the only boy who'd ever expressed interest in me was reedy-voiced Alex, who'd been taken out of our rough-and-tumble comprehensive and sent to a private boys' school shortly afterward. Chris, on the other hand, was high-school royalty—one of those people referred to by both first and last name, as if calling him plain Chris conveyed a lack of respect. It would never have occurred to me to make a move on him, mainly because if I'd given it any real thought, I'd have come up against the knowledge that while I cared about him—about his parents' divorce, his university applications and the fate of a history essay he'd spent weeks on—I didn't crave him, and I didn't feel the queasy thrill that I felt looking at the boy who would eventually succeed him. We had a sweetly earnest friendship, Chris and I; we just weren't sure where the physical bit fitted in.

On a sheet of lined writing paper, he wrote me a letter that I still have, though its cobalt ink has paled into the past and his oddly loopy *t*'s (what would a handwriting expert say?) make it hard to read. In between pledges of friendship are regrets about feeling inept and being overly cautious. I count it as my first and only love letter, even though it was written after he'd "broken up" with me. That had occurred as we rode the bus back from a party in a club where it was too loud to talk and too dark to see. He needed to focus more on his studies, he told me, meaning that I was dumped not for another girl but for Bismarck. He seemed to mean it, and spent the remaining term and a half hidden away in the library.

It was pride that he'd wooed in me and pride that he wounded.

That night, I cried. The following afternoon, I went out and bought myself a scarlet lipstick, the founding item in a cache of breakup, buck-up buys that would swell to include everything from impossible shoes to airline tickets. Chris and I parted as virgins, but we'd lost our innocence in other ways. He'd learned that you can like a girl too much, and that showing her you like her even a little can sometimes wreck your chances. And me? I'd gained a clearer sense of whom it was that I might be in the eyes of boys. Over the coming eighteen months or so, I would winnow my wardrobe of outsized garments down to a single giant black jumper, felted with wear. I clung on to it for years, retreating into its moth-eaten expanse whenever my self-image wavered—whenever I flunked a student essay or, later, filed an article I wasn't pleased with, or whenever some boy broke up with me.

Asked whom we dress for, most of us will answer, with unhesitating piety, for ourselves, but if our personal sense of worth is our ultimate concern, we are also dressing for an audience—dressing to blend in, to stand out, to impress. That audience is not made up of men. After all, just think about the times you've gone shopping with a straight man. What has he picked out? I remember one years-ago Sunday morning, a man who briefly filled the role of boyfriend asked me whether I'd consider wearing an anklet. We were camped out on his bed, surrounded by papers and bagels and smoked salmon. An anklet? He broke off reading to clamp inky fingers around my ankle as if showing me how alluring it might look. He'd won me round by being able to make me laugh at almost anything, but at that particular moment, his eyes betrayed rapt seriousness.

Another time, another man cajoled me into a clothes shop. We'd been shopping together and bought plenty for him, nothing for me. He would turn out to be a bolter, but like so many serial bolters, he began by being overwhelmingly, anxiously attentive. It was as if he sensed me keeping my distance, resisting that jointly decided purchase. So there we were, he and I, rifling through rails of women's clothes. Maybe it's a weirdness on my part, but I have to know someone well before I'll go clothes shopping with them. On that particular day, I had no intention of buying anything, but the man at my side didn't let this stop him, especially when he spotted the peasant smocks (remember that summer when they were suddenly everywhere?).

"Wouldn't you wear this?" he asked, eagerly tugging at the sleeve of a balloonlike garment, sequined and tasseled, that may have been a dress or a tunic or perhaps a generously proportioned skirt, the kind in which lusty milkmaids galumph on fragrant pastures. I could almost smell the alpine herbs. It was a glimpse of another's interior life—a life in which I, at least for a few months, played the part of a woman I would never have recognized.

It happened again with a man I'd thought knew me far better, a man who has become a recurring motif in my romantic mishaps. The Beau, I'll call him, in the hope that it'll give you a sense of his eccentric panache and dapper wardrobe, and the fact that he has a couple of decades on me. A still-boyish American, he is a devoted amateur yachtsman, fond of Europe's gentler waters. Though he tries to hide it, his background is in computing, and when he was in his thirties and forties, his life was firmly rooted on dry land. He is hazy about the details, but at some point, he struck a deal that enabled him to cast off for good. Now he makes only occasional forays ashore, calling me out of the blue from one of his old urban stamping grounds. We've drifted close to getting involved over the years, and back then were in a gray area, hurrying through New York's SoHo on a gelid January evening, when he stopped abruptly in front of a shop window.

Did I mention that it was cold? It was icicle, blizzard, grounded-flights cold—cold enough for us to have skipped a party the evening before, staying in to watch DVDs and feel awkward with each other rather than brave a few riverside blocks. And it was far, far too cold for window-shopping, but there he stood, smiling up at a dummy sporting a tiny power suit, miniskirted and nipped in at the bosom. She was dressed for neither the meteorological nor the fashion moment.

"That would look amazing on you," he said, muffled by layers of scarf and coat and a Tibetan hat in blinding neon shades, purchased in a shoe store earlier on out of frozen desperation (shoes they knew, hats they did not).

So no, we're not dressing for men, but we're not dressing for women, either. We're dressing *against* them. It's other women who are most likely to clock the cut of your new top or the delicate shade of the raspberry pullover that you fell for despite its scary price tag, but there's often an edge to their praise—a competitive edge that has to do with sex. We may not be prepared to wear anklets, but we'll gladly clobber the competition, flaunting our sexuality with a swaggering menace. After all, isn't there something aggressive in the scanty costume of reality TV starlets out on the town?

They are an extreme example, I hear you protest, and I'd agree were it not for my attitude toward the two sales assistants back in the clothes shop on this September afternoon. I may have the power of the customer here, but they are both younger than me, and far prettier, too. I'd rather not acknowledge it, but I can't help myself—

I'm absurdly glad that in between wrapping all those bulky woolens, they have to deal with a slithery slip of silk, a budget-busting wisp of a blouse that I've thrown in on a whim. Watching me watch them, my sister catches my victory smile, onto me right away. Is it even chaste? More so than you'd think. Its buttons button to the neck and its sleeves, though dainty, cover my shoulders.

If it seems strange that having made such a personal, private decision, I'm seeking to solidify it by altering my outward appearance—by trading a lace-trimmed camisole for a turtleneck jumper—consider this: clothing is our way of signaling to the world who we are, or who we'd like to be. As such, it has its own language, and if we let it, it'll do the talking for us. As actress Emma Watson has since told a *Daily Mail* journalist, "I find the whole concept of being 'sexy' embarrassing and confusing. If I do a photo-shoot people desperately want to change me—dye my hair blonde, pluck my eyebrows, give me a fringe. Then there's the choice of clothes. I know everyone wants a picture of me in a mini-skirt. But that's not me."

It's not quite that we are what we wear, but what we wear becomes us—it becomes us even when it doesn't suit us. Rummage through your own wardrobe. There are your skinny jeans—not skinny-cut, perhaps, but the ones that fit you only at your leanest, meaning that you walk taller whenever you step out in them. Then there's the dress that makes you hold your shoulders just so in order to keep its silky spaghetti straps from slipping. The way you hold your shoulders changes your posture, lending you allure even on an evening when you'd rather be slouched in front of the telly. With your dress leading the way, you're cast as another woman, sending signals rippling out ahead of you and subtly changing the way you feel in your own skin.

If I'd wanted to, I could have logged on and ordered from a range of ModesTees. Manufactured by a company based in Utah, they are designed to be worn beneath garments whose cut seems too revealing—or whose fabric too sheer, as is the case with my blouse. The same company also offers a dress line called Sweet Innocence—satin, jersey and chiffon numbers that might at first glance have come from any mail-order clothing catalog. Look again, and you'll note that their skirts all cover the knee, none is sleeveless and the necklines are high enough to conceal the wearer's collarbone. There are bathing suits, too, which boast "complete bottom coverage" and come with optional skirts, just in case.

It's easy to mock such endeavors. As liberated women, we are rightly suspicious of anyone, male or female, who seeks to cloak our form. And who wouldn't want to cheer on the women of Afghanistan for wearing heels beneath their burkas as they pick their way along potholed roads? Back in the 1730s, the English letter writer Lady Mary Wortley Montagu captured a timeless spirit of rebellion in her satirical couplet "Summary of Lord Lyttelton's Advice": "Be plain in dress, and sober in your diet; In short, my deary, kiss me and be quiet."

Its skewed latter-day realization is neatly summed up in modesty-nik Wendy Shalit's latest book, *Girls Gone Mild,* with a deftly chosen quote from *Bratz: Babyz the Movie:* "You've gotta look hotter than hot! Show what you've got!" Most of the film's target audience, remember, are hardly out of diapers themselves.

Yet, as fashionista Elise Vallee revealed in *The Well-Dressed Woman's Do's and Don'ts,* the "exaggerated display of chest, and especially of back" was passé even in 1925. By the time Cole Porter's musical *Anything Goes* debuted on Broadway in 1934, a glimpse of stocking was a distinctly olden-days thrill.

We continue to think of sartorial rebellion as being all about stripping down, but while today's dare-to-bare designs merely emphasize the female form, historically the clothing that shocks most have been styles that muddle gender distinctions. That garb also has the headiest ambitions, donned by women who have sought to claim the privileges and opportunities of the male world. "Dress is a small thing, among the littlest," the virgin martyr Joan of Arc said. She got that wrong—of all her maverick misdeeds, it was her cross-dressing that most enraged her English captors.

Women's clothing remains a battlefield. At its root are two contradictory notions—a male desire to control female sexuality and its threatening fertility, coupled with the admission that they cannot even control their own sexuality, and that the burden of keeping their appetites in check resides with women, whose duty it is to vanish lest they inflame male passion. Of course, most garments intended to contain women's sexuality end up drawing attention to it. At their most extreme, they become fetish objects, like chastity belts or bound feet.

In light of such charged discourse, my hopes for my own new clothes are modest indeed: merely that they will prove roomy enough for me to figure out what kind of an image I'd like to project; and to learn to do as stern Ms. Phelps counseled and characterize my clothes rather than have them characterize me.

As it turns out, that blouse is about to come into its own, because I have a date. You might wonder what I'm up to, heading off to meet a man just a few weeks into a year-long attempt at chastity. It's partly that I'm still trying to push Jake from my mind. It's been almost two months since I last saw him—six weeks and five days to be precise, and I really need to lose count. But the truth is, my vow hasn't yet sunk in. Though it seems to be going against the spirit of it, I feel like I need to test it in order to prove its existence.

As the date nears, my resolve falters. Is it their artificiality that makes dates such chilly experiences? While Americans have created an entire rulebook of dating mores, we Brits can't seem to get the hang of them. Our national traits just aren't suited to the format. In the formal, forced setting of a date, our self-deprecation, for instance, self-detonates.

Actually, my worst so far has been with an American. An older man whose job involved organizing vast sums of money and large groups of difficult people, he had planned it perfectly. We met on the South Bank and went to see some neon art—works whose medium lent them a seamy glamour, perfect for light-starved midwinter. As we paused dutifully before each exhibit, I realized that though I'd been seated beside this man at dinner parties over the years, I didn't know him at all.

It could have been thrilling, that flash of knowledge, but instead it threw me into a kind of panic as we moved on to dinner. The restaurant was a sophisticated staple overlooking the Thames, which flowed dark and glossy through the night. He barraged me with questions, ensuring that I glimpsed not a chink of what might lie beyond his own carefully positioned social armor. Without quite understanding what I was doing, I responded in kind, going into charm overdrive and setting up a barrier between us as I rehearsed for him all the cute tales I've ever told on a date. It was as if I were sketching a stylized stand-in me. By the time he dropped me off with the swiftest of kisses on my cheek, I felt like I'd spent the evening with a hologram of myself—a neon-bright and wildly unfaithful self-portrait.

The odd thing is that months later, long after I'd spun a funny story from the date's quietly crushing details (he'd actually dropped me at a bus stop rather than drive ten minutes more to my house), I heard via a mutual friend that he'd figured I was already involved with someone. Maybe he was just trying to be retroactively kind, but if not, what had given him that impression?

It must have been what I was wearing, I decided. I'd come straight from the office in a cashmere sweater, snug-fitting but unmistakably turtlenecked, and a skirt whose dove-gray velvet swirled out when twirled on a dance floor but fell drably to my knees in any other scenario—picking anxiously at my food, say. I'd looked forward to that date—or so I told myself. But a less gullibly romantic part of my brain must have computed what I knew of him—his relationship track record, his age, his crowd—and decided that this was not such a good idea. That was the part that guided my hand as I picked out the day's—and the evening's—outfit in the half-light of a December morning.

The neon date is very much on my mind as I prepare to leave the office and head out to this other. Seeing me scoop books from my desk, a colleague begins to ask me what I'll wear, swerving tactfully as she realizes that I'll be wearing exactly this: a slightly weary smile, charcoal trousers—the wide-legged kind that make for dramatic exits—and a black sweater with, yes, a turtleneck. What my colleague doesn't know is that I'm also wearing the new blouse, a sheath of sheer silk, hidden from sight but slippery against my skin.

My date's name is Mark and he is a friend of a friend. We met a short while ago at a lunch designed for that very purpose, and having passed each other's preliminary tests—the sidelong glances and gentle probing—we're now venturing out on our own. Mark is about my age. He is smart, attentive and good-looking in a smooth-edged, calming way. When your eyes rest on his face, they truly rest—there is nothing to jar in his perfectly proportioned features. He is also a marine biologist—an aquatic Indiana Jones, a sly voice in my head whispers. Think how good he'd look in a wet suit! it urges. As I slide into a seat opposite him in a low-key Turkish restaurant, I can't help thinking precisely that, though I also notice that my body registers not a flicker of curiosity.

Perhaps that's what is missing—that twinge of physical inquisitiveness. Listen in, and you'll hear me and Mark chat-chat-chatting away. You won't hear any awkwardness, but you'll feel it, even with the waiters zipping back and forth between your table and ours. It's the fluency of our chat that gives us away: we're terrified of the silence.

What would follow if we let that silence be awhile, if the space between us were to fill for just a few minutes with the clink and scrape of other people's meals? Would it grow chasmic or would it pull us closer together? Might silence and distance be the ultimate test of compatibility? Imagine an alternative speed-dating in which people sit wordlessly opposite their would-be mates, listening so hard for cosmic reverberations humming between them that they miss the buzzer telling them it's time to switch seats.

This isn't a blind date, but it is beginning to feel short-sighted. In our determination to prove to ourselves and to each other that we aren't on anything that remotely resembles a date, we almost succeed. By the time the meze is served—finger-friendly food that suggests sharing more than just falafel and dips—our chatty chatter has homed in on a single safe topic: work. It's as if I'm dining with an out-of-town colleague. "Sex is like eating and eating is like sex," Casanova said. There's a lot left on our plates when our waiter comes to ask if we'd like coffee.

Afterward, I'm resigning myself to a meandering bus ride home when I spot a taxi—not exactly an ascetic choice, but its illuminated FOR HIRE sign is enough of an omen for me to raise my hand. Mark lets me drop him at the nearest tube station, and as we pull up at a red light, he leans over to peck me on the cheek, simultaneously reaching into his wallet for a donation with one hand while opening the door with the other. I'm still telling him not to bother about the fare as he dives out into three streams of barely stationary traffic. Engines rev impatiently amid sheeny metal and angry taillights, then the door bangs shut. It's a silly, funny stunt. Alone in the cab, half listening for the dreaded sound of screeching brakes, I reflect that though they may not dress for it, men play roles, too. And what has my own been this evening, on the occasion of my first chaste date? You'd have to check with Mark, but dusty librarian seems likely.

Back home, I peel off my sweater and there it is, the little black shirt. Unbuttoning it and shaking it out, I see that it's worn-looking— crumpled beneath the arms, its dainty collar tugged out of shape by the turtleneck. But it hasn't been wasted, because as I sat making small talk and peering over invisible pince-nez, I knew it was there and was thankful.

The truth is, I was on a date whose benign pleasantness was also the source of its bleakness. Mark wasn't Jake, and unless it's him sitting across the table, I'm not interested. Chastity will be easy, I think, and at the same time my heart, still bruised, sinks a little. In a culture in which we're all supposed to be wanting and wanted—in which fashion, in particular, is advertised by models whose poses mime constant desire—I feel like I've lost some crucial part of myself. What am I thinking as my first month nears its close? Truthfully, it's not what you'd expect. My worry is not that I won't make it to the end, but that I'll make it to the end with this absence of ardor intact.

Have I felt this way before? I don't think so, though it's true that in the past I would probably have listened to that campy advice to get myself over one man by wriggling beneath the comforting weight of another. Invariably, the recovery fling would be with a man from my past, one with whom I had enough shared history to draw on that I could conceal my absence of feeling from the both of us. In those instances, sex was my solution to the panicky feeling of not wanting. It was as if I hoped lust would rub off on me as we scrambled beneath the sheets. Not feeling wanted is bad enough, but not feeling want is arguably more unnerving.

That impulse-buy blouse is a talisman of something that I need to know is still there. We're not meant to believe as much, but deep down, I think that for most of us, allure remains bound up with desirability. Coco Chanel insisted that elegance was not about putting on a new dress, that it was something you radiated from within, but when it comes to allure, it often seems conferred by the attention of others—something that rests in the validation of a lingering gaze or a door held open. We can accentuate it with swooping necklines and sheer fabrics, but we're always waiting for another to confirm it. It's a lot to burden a wisp of fabric with, but in tuning out the brassy clamor of who I'm meant to be and taking the chaste option and wearing it hidden and close to me, I feel as if I'm becoming reacquainted with my own femininity. And there's something else, too: I'm reminded of how thrilling the hidden can be, of the power of holding a secret that you can choose to reveal or not reveal. There's a word for this, a forgotten word: *modesty*.

Meanwhile, to the outside world, my vow seems to have swathed me in a giant, mystical black turtleneck. Black turtlenecks are the uniform of French intellectuals, of rebels whose heads are full of ideas that spill over onto the streets, volatile as Molotov cocktails. A man leaped from a barely stationary car to escape me this evening—has my vow made me dangerous, too? It's an enticing thought.

FOUR

October OR *Brief Encounters*

> It's woman's spirit and mood a man has to
> stimulate in order to make sex interesting.
> The real lover is the man who can thrill you
> by touching your head or smiling into your
> eyes or just staring into space.
>
> —Marilyn Monroe

At the start of October, my new wardrobe and I are packed off to the continent to cover a trade conference. The word *continent* makes this dank, nicotine-fingered northern European city sound far more glamorous than it will ever be. Even *trade conference* seems to be overselling the experience. Yet one aspect of this trip is rather too exciting.

As a last-minute delegate, I had to look hard to find a room, and while everyone else is billeted in one of several towering chain hotels, I'm staying in a smaller place, ominously close to the railway station. Clearly, this establishment once rented rooms by the hour, and a sleek makeover hasn't made it coy about its past. Its bar is open twenty-four hours a day, and you expect the lobby clock to read three A.M. even at nine o'clock on a brisk Monday morning, perhaps because of the perpetually low lighting and music that is so bass-heavy you register it more as a pulsing beat in your chest than as a sound.

When people ask me where I'm staying, I don't mention any of this—all I need do is dangle my key before them. In lieu of a key ring there swings an enormous braided bauble. Pendulous is the word—obscenely pendulous. Mostly it has elicited laughter and knowingly raised eyebrows, though I've glimpsed the beginnings of a blush or two. Either way, without knowing about my vow, no one can fully appreciate the irony of that bauble nor the mocking delights that it unlocks—the silky coverlet, the cream suede headboard, the dusky furniture. Even the floor seems to cry out for action, carpeted in a decadent checkerboard pattern that intimates Jacobean excess—infidelities and revenge, poison-lined robes and spiked goblets.

For the best part of a week, I wake in this improbable setting, peering in at a breakfast of cheese and meat before setting out to traipse moving walkways. I seem to be forever trying to get from one identical exhibition hall to another. I don't know how many miles of moving walkways there are, but to give you just a hint, I manage to conduct an entire twenty-minute interview without treading more than three paces on solid ground. Occasionally I'll glimpse friends and colleagues—the bright smile of one, already fixed and fading by day two, the woebegone slouch of another, camouflaged in a gray shirt. It's an oddly exhausting experience, striding along a conveyor belt, especially with so little in the passing scenery to suggest that you're actually going anywhere. This is how my days are spent.

The nights are longer than all the moving walkways put together and almost as disorientating. It turns out that the only way to shut off after a ten-hour stretch of talking shop is to stand shoulder-to-shoulder in a hot, din-filled bar, drinking strong drinks and shouting shop. But another kind of dialogue fills the air here, too. As the crush packs us closer together and the drinks make us sloppy about our bodies, sharp elbows press into soft waists and bosoms heave against backs. With voices growing hoarse, lips brush ears saying far more than their drowned-out words could.

Is the particular trade relevant? Probably not, though I should explain that these professionals trade in stories. They are here to oil the wheels of commerce and to listen out for a good tale or two, and they know that the fizzle of attraction can play a part in both. To my newly chaste ears, the sexual undercurrent is deafening. Am I the only one who hears it? Would I have heard it ordinarily, or simply been swept along? While it's mostly without intent and will go no farther than the bar, like the decor back at my hotel, it feels too much.

Of course, that decor is a tease—it cannot mask the generic hotel bleakness that sneaks up on you even when you're in a hot resort with a lover to pinch the second pillow-chocolate from. You may not notice it, but it will be there, lurking under the bed, waiting to jump out once you're all packed up and are giving the room a last glance over for stray belongings. It's a haunting presence that has only ever been an absence—the absence created by people just passing through, people like you. Held at a distance by my vow, I can appreciate the humanity in all that barroom flirtation. Flailing and ungainly, or else knowing, too smooth, it nonetheless represents a kind of reaching out, and uses only the language that seems to be expected of us, here especially. After all, everyone knows what happens at conferences away from home—sex is what happens.

This newfound clarity doesn't exempt me from those same impulses. As I ride the endless moving walkways, a man has been flitting in and out of my thoughts. Each evening, I catch myself looking for him in the bar. We met on day two. I was due to interview a woman with a dazzling CV and had arrived too early, pitching up while she was still in a meeting. Just as I turned to leave, she gestured for me to stay and take a seat. On her other side was a guy who looked my age, and maybe that's it—maybe it's just that being a little younger than her gave us something in common, making him seem like someone I could talk to in real life, away from the strip lighting and carpet tiles.

Paradoxically, he also seemed like precisely the kind I would never have noticed prevow. He is the archetypal quiet guy in the corner, and a few months back I simply wouldn't have heard him. Though I was trying to focus on my interviewee, I glimpsed an occasional flash of fair hair, and hands made for something outdoorsy rather than twiddling a pen. He says little, but his voice, when he does speak, is warmed by an accent—American, Southern. I tell myself he's just a nice idea to fall asleep to—that if I sense some physical connection, it's on the level of kinship rather than anything sexual.

Back in the bar, all those lingering looks and brushed fingertips crescendo with the closing-night party. On that evening, I make a pit stop at my train-station boudoir and change into a dress. Though it might not pass for one of ModesTee's Sweet Innocence designs, it is skimming rather than fitted, with a neckline that barely reveals my collarbone.

The party turns out to be just another trade party, albeit with music and dimmer lighting, but the night unfurls with a sideways flourish. I'm with a crowd that includes the Quiet Guy, and on the way there, the taxi takes us far out into the suburbs and beyond, flashing past a forest and out onto an industrial estate where music throbs from an abandoned warehouse. The driver has his radio turned up loud, and in between bursts of foreign-language chat, a British singer belts out a number so dirtily soulful it sounds naked.

Afterward, sitting once again in the bar, we drift in a huddle toward that unreal time when you're too tired to do anything but stay awake. In between trancelike silences, we trade truths about ourselves—telltale details disguised as inanities, like what we'd eat right now if we were anywhere other than this dumpy conference town. Pancakes is my answer, and it's the Quiet Guy's, too.

With every passing half hour, our band of revelers thins. Eventually, it is just the Quiet Guy and me. Perhaps we should have persuaded one of the others to stay? Not that we need a chaperone, it's just that in some situations, the story seems to take over. The time and the place and the setting exert a narrative power that becomes irresistible. I can see how it might happen even here. We'd wander back to his hotel to check out the breakfast buffet, only we'd be too early, or we'd hit restaurant rush hour. For some reason or other, we'd be forced to retreat to his room. There we'd be, and there the bed would be, and often, one plus one plus a bed equals—well, one thing only.

I'm fairly certain that my vow is safe, that I wouldn't let things get that far, but can't help noting how much I'm enjoying playing out this scenario in my head. Of course, I probably wouldn't be here at all were it not for the vow. Those Quiet Guy traits that I'm finding so entrancing right now—that hint of reticence, the thoughtfulness that offsets his swift smile—would before have been too subtle to register with me. They are of a different frequency. I'd have been carried along on that other current of deafeningly obvious sex appeal.

Apart from us two, there is no one else in the bar—until suddenly there is. Just like that (and just when I've silently acknowledged the flimsiness of my resolve), the most attractive man I've seen in a long, long time appears. A chaperone? Not exactly. He has the kind of coloring that can't be faked—buttermilk skin, golden-syrup locks falling across a coffee gaze. It's as if he's been snipped straight from my dreams of love and breakfast.

With a thrill, I realize that he is looking right at me. For a moment, I'm sure he's about to step over—perhaps he knows the Quiet Guy? But no, he's gone. Except that here he is again, slowly lapping the big room beyond the bar, where it seems to have grown so late it's early—early enough for waiters to be shuffling chairs into a breakfast formation and throwing white tablecloths over surfaces that just moments ago were cluttered with lipstick-kissed glasses. Did he lose something here earlier on? Again he fixes me with that look, and as it happens a third time, a fourth, I begin to feel embarrassed.

It's less a look than a stare, the kind of stare that I've no idea what to do with in my chaste state. Once, I'd have stared boldly back, but now I'm flustered, altogether less certain. Irrationally, I can't help feeling that if the bar had been full, his gaze would have been diluted along the way. Thrown through the empty air, its impact is way too strong. It's tequila-slammer strong—with a whiskey float. Though I'm sunk in a chintzy chair with just a dreggy ice cube in my glass, a wave of giddiness passes over me.

There is a dreamlike clarity to the scene. Everything is vivid and yet I'm powerless to do anything unless I wake up, but I'm as awake as I will ever be at this hour of this strange week, so instead I sit tight and listen to the Quiet Guy. He's not so quiet, it turns out; he just happens to think awhile before responding.

Meanwhile the other guy—my usual type if you flipped his coloring from fair to dark—struts in and out of my line of vision, flagrant in his sexy dishevelment and the increasing boldness of that stare. I'd wonder whether I didn't know him were he not so very attractive. No woman could forget a man this delicious. Not even my newly married friend Caroline, who has materialized at my shoulder.

"That guy . . . ," she whispers, twinkly-eyed. "He is *hot!*"

She is from California, which means that she can make pro-
nouncements like that without sounding as if she's stepped off the
set of a high-school miniseries. And she's right, of course, so the
next time we make eye contact, I say something—nothing plucky or
spunky or memorable, just a "hi," croaked out in party-worn tones.
"Hi," he says back, and wanders over to sit on the arm of my chair.
My chaste self feels like leaping up but I haven't the energy. I introduce everyone and there they both are, he and the Quiet Guy caught
side by side in the same frame. It's hard not to be drawn to the newcomer. He's wearing a sheepskin jacket, for heaven's sake—a man
who dresses in animal pelts and seems to carry the sun on his skin.

He is Israeli, it turns out, and, like every other Hebrew speaker
I've ever met, he knows all about my biblical name. Unlike those
others, he doesn't smile and give me its meaning ("my delight is in
her"—particularly ironic given the quest I'm embarked upon, but
still, to hear it from his mouth!). Instead, he frowns and repeats it
incredulously. "Hephzibah? It is like being called . . . Ethel in English," he says, shaking his head sadly before delivering the final
blow: "It is an old-people name."

Well, I *am* an old person in relation to him. I'm not sure how the
conversation arrived so swiftly at this point, but he has just revealed
that he is all of twenty-six years old. Four years younger than me, a
year younger than my younger sister. "You're not," I say, laughing
confidently. "You can't be, you have to be *thirty*-six."

"How old do you want me to be?" he asks, and instantly it feels
as if I'm the one who's been doing the running here, scoping him out
as he mooched around the bar, minding his own business. Could it
actually have been that way? Perhaps my hotel digs are rubbing off
on me. In my defense, he really does look thirty-six, though maybe

the hour has added a decade to each of us. But twenty-six he is, and as if proof were needed, just as he is jokingly trying to persuade me to visit him back home next week, and not a minute later, his phone rings.

"Yes?" he answers, cooler than cool. I wonder if it's a girlfriend. There must be several. "I'm in the bar. . . . No. . . . Yes, but the flight's not until nine-thirty. *No,* I'll be back in time. Okay. . . . Okay, Dad, I'm *coming.*"

The evening ends a little after dawn, with a margarita for breakfast. After ninety minutes' sleep and long airport delays, I'm finally away. At the other end, milling by the baggage carousel, I almost walk straight into a long-ago ex—anklet man. It feels like poetic justice for having wavered back in the bar.

We like to think that people come in types, and it's our "type" that we wrestle with throughout our dating years. Initially, it's all about honing him. We like our lovers broad-shouldered, we tell ourselves. They have to be square of jaw and smoldering of gaze, lazy-tongued and quick-thinking. But rules are made to be broken, and what begins as a quest for positives becomes about negatives—it becomes a process of elimination. Lanky men didn't work out, so how about a sturdier type, someone more grounded? The intellectuals were angst-ridden, so what about a chef or a landscape gardener? Or perhaps our mothers were right all along, there really is nothing wrong with a nice doctor—but does not being wrong make him right, and if so, how right is right enough?

Before you know it, you're stuck on a seesaw of remedy dating, prescribing each successive relationship in an attempt to cancel out the one that's gone before. Eventually it is impossible to tell the symptoms from the side effects—and yes, it's come to this, you're thinking about relationships as if they were seasonal snuffles, something to be endured.

A short while ago, my friend Melissa got married. She made the happiest bride any of us had ever seen, but during the reception, she reminded me and some of her school friends that while she and her husband of five hours had been smitten at first sight, she'd had a reservation, a big one. He had dark hair, you see, while she traditionally liked her men fair. I wasn't the only one who felt suddenly jaded: how was it that our friend had weathered a good decade of dating and only now had to surrender such a fairy-tale stipulation? I thought of The Group. During the same period, we'd watched one another chuck out a whole range of fundamental requirements, from a guy's actually liking us to his being single. Our relationships had become a version of that team-building exercise where you're in a sinking hot-air balloon and have to figure out what to ditch next— except that there is no team to build, we're in there on our own. Yet here was Melissa, beaming mischievously at herself for having ended up with the brown-haired prince rather than the yellow-haired one.

Pinning down my own type is tricky—that's his first characteristic. I seem to pick the ones who really do not want to be pinned. The fly-by-nights, the cads, the all-round rotters. They've come in a baffling array of shapes and sizes, though they've all been older than me—some older than others; others much, much older than some.

But perhaps all this profiling is simply paving the way for someone to come along and astonish us. For someone who is so resolutely not our type that we're defenseless against their charms. Quiet Guy, for instance. Since returning from that conference, I've received a series of e-mails from him. They started out strictly work-related— only fitting for a chaste girl like myself—but with each new note we have drifted a little closer toward the personal. He tells me about his sister and her new twins. He acquires a dog. A coziness creeps into our correspondence. It offers the friendly warmth I'd been searching for that week—the warmth I might have been tempted to seek in the arms of the syrup-haired dreamboat, if it hadn't been for my vow and his slender years. This is, in its way, a revelation—the quiet guy in the corner, the one who, in my world of alternative circumstances, I would scarcely have noticed. "Talk soon," he signs off each time, and I get to thinking what it would be like to actually pick up the phone and hear his honeyed drawl at the other end.

"What about your vow?" my sister demands as soon as I mention having met him. I'm careful to describe him in neutral terms, slipping him into the conversation between details of conference-center catering and the weather, but she knows me too well. She's right, of course—whatever this is, I need to snap out of it. He's so far away, off in Los Angeles, that it feels like a safely chaste dalliance, but still, it is becoming something to torture myself with. Besides, while I can try to deceive myself about my own feelings, I can't disguise his, which I'm certain are purely platonic. After all, he didn't know about my vow—what was to stop him from trying to instigate something back in that bar? Except what if he really is interested and just likes to take things at a more leisurely pace—the pace of his conversation, say?

I know, I'm just trying to cushion myself from his lack of interest—which shouldn't matter to me right now anyway—yet it's true that when a man doesn't make his move swiftly, we think it odd. Two very different friends of my sister both found themselves between the sheets with men who, for no obvious reason, stopped at foreplay. Once was sweet, twice unusual, thrice downright bizarre. The one girl is a vixen, at ease with her own voluptuousness; the other carries off primness with such assurance it becomes chic. Their reactions to this novel turn of events were identical: they panicked. They hadn't been spurned, not exactly, but it shook their confidence. Though both anxiously solicited advice from friends, neither wanted to ask the men themselves. If the roles were reversed—if it had been the women resisting—would it have seemed so odd? Probably—certainly by the third occasion—but not quite to the same extent. Once would have been expected, twice almost coquettish, thrice simply irritating. In liberating ourselves from the slyly constructed myth that women are not sexual beings—that, as one Dr. O. A. Wall summarized in 1932, "A well-bred woman does not seek carnal gratification, and she is usually apathetic to sexual pleasures"—we have imprisoned men in a counterpart belief that they are hypersexual, constantly on the lookout for carnal relief—or, if not constantly, at least every fifty-two seconds.

In this particular instance, it is the fact that nothing happened between us that makes Quiet Guy such a potent figure in my imagination. Stuck on that romantic seesaw, you begin to feel like it's your duty to test every lingering possibility. The sad truth is that sometimes, at our loneliest, we fall not for this person or that but for the image of ourselves that they project onto us—a smarter, prettier, better-loved soul. Of course, once tested, it turns out to be just another mirage.

Quiet Guy isn't exceptional. Looking back, it's the men I haven't slept with whom I remember most fondly. I don't mean the ones who've spurned me, though there have been plenty, and we all know there's nothing quite like the cold shoulder for making the heart grow fonder. No, I mean those almost-affairs, the guys I came tantalizingly close to kissing, or the men I kissed but for one reason or another didn't go any further with. However great the sex was with other men, it's they who can still tug at my heart years later, who'll bring a secretive smile to my face if ever their name crops up over a glass of wine with girlfriends. "Whatever happened to . . . ?" one of The Group will ask, and for a moment I'll be lost to the conversation, off pursuing a coulda-shoulda-woulda alternative reality. Looking up, I'll see knowing smiles on their faces—we all have those men, men who belong to unfinished stories.

Sexless narratives can take their place in the realm of make-believe, alongside all the romantic notions that we doggedly cling to, often in perfect defiance of experience and logic. "The One," for instance—how can we believe in him when we've been confident of having found him so many times before?

"Tell me," a man once whispered to me in the dark, "tell me your fantasy." His words were hot and his stubble rough as his hands sent shivery ripples coursing from my earlobes down to my toes. To help me, he sketched some scenarios. I take a wrong turn in a boys' school and wind up in the showers, surrounded by young men. Or we're at a black-tie dinner together, and slip out into a dew-washed garden, where he hoists up my dress and begins to unbutton his fly—except that it isn't that simple. In fact it's very complicated, involving all sorts of buttons and zips and suspenders. Predictable stuff, but then that is the curious thing: pressed to reveal our innermost desires, our revelations turn out to draw on a very limited imaginative vocabulary. Psychotherapist Brett Kahr proved as much when he set about compiling his mammoth study of British sexual fantasies, *Sex and the Psyche:* our narratives are so personal, and yet at the same time so prosaically impersonal.

So what was my fantasy? The one I really wanted to share—the one that would surely have shocked that man right out of my bed—was that he might be someone who loved me. But it seemed just too kinky, so instead I mumbled about shipwrecks and desert islands, trying to muffle my sniggers with the sheet.

As I reflect on this, I'm lying flat on my back, being maneuvered into a series of embarrassing, lip-bitingly painful positions. The air is tense with exertion, laced with the scents of sweat and feet and the musky incense meant to mask them. These are not positions I'm supposed to be assuming. I'm supposed to be in my weekly beginner's Pilates class, but this? This is yoga, and it most certainly is not for beginners. I've been running late the whole week, and all those missing minutes have added up to make me very late indeed for the Sunday evening class. Arriving in a red-faced fluster, I must have misheard the studio number down at the front desk.

The natural thing would have been to slip out as soon as I'd realized my error, but for some reason, I have not done this. Our instructor is as bendy as a pipe cleaner, but listen and you'll hear a steely note in each of her breathy commands.

"Swing your legs over your head. Place your forearms flat on the mat. Now walk your body up in an arc. Hold it, hold it. And . . ."

It is torture. To exit at this stage would be admitting failure, and even though staying proves the exact same thing, I've lost the will to protest any of it.

". . . relax."

It has been a long weekend back in London. Last night I met my friend Victoria for a drink. I was her bridesmaid earlier on in the spring. A small wedding, she'd promised—a small New York wedding. Another friend had tipped me off to the contradiction immediately. "A small New York wedding? No. No, no, no." She was right: Victoria's guest list was intimate, but it was a great big production. From the moment I accepted my role, our friendship became strained. A full week before the big day, I flew out to New York together with the best man and a mutual friend, as instructed. While she was staying with her parents, we rented an apartment, which turned out fine but didn't seem that way to begin with.

"I can't let you out here," our cab driver said. He had spent the journey humming along to a piano concerto, breaking off to tell us that he'd been to London and loved our Indian restaurants. But this was Manhattan, his patch, and he didn't like the address we'd given him. "You're sure you wrote it down right? Because those buildings—see there?—those are the projects." I had written it down right—we were staying on the fringes of some project-type housing, but Lincoln Center was right around the corner. From these budget digs, we ventured out each day on high-end wedding errands. Victoria's mother spoiled us with couture dresses, killer heels and dancing lessons. Her father kept our spirits up with good wines and sharp jokes, but with the big day looming, everyone was flagging.

Somehow I was drafted to accompany the soon-to-be bride and her groom down to City Hall, where I stood with them in line after line as their papers accrued the stamps and signatures needed to become a license to wed—window one, window two, window three. At window seven, the person standing on the other side of the counter could actually officiate, and proclaim you husband and wife there and then. Weren't they in the least bit tempted? I know I would have been, after a week of having to make decisions about everything from where to seat tricky relatives to which side of the plate the green beans should be placed on.

Naturally, everything about that City Hall experience was set up for two. I was in a room filled with happy couples—happy couples looking anxiously ahead and checking their watches, happy couples worrying about where they'd left the car parked, happy couples snapping at each other about the placement of green beans. Still, if ever I was going to have a meltdown about my single status, that huge room filled with its two-by-two lines would have been the place. It's a measure of the craziness of that week that I didn't envy them, not a bit. There was just one moment when I registered a little pang: the love hearts.

That great municipal room was set in the inner sanctum of a building so fortified it's a wonder I was let in as a spare extra. Yet at shoulder height, scrawled in ballpoint pen all over its walls, were the kinds of love hearts that you see on tree trunks and in school notebooks: "Scott 'n' Linda," "Annette luvs Juan." Most carried dates, and none was older than four or five months. The room must have been repainted regularly in the full knowledge that each fresh coat of paint merely created more space for the lovers—love scrawled on love scrawled on love. Even the City Hall bureaucrats had a soft spot for it.

Miraculously, my friendship with the bride survived the wedding, but relations had grown only more difficult in its wake. Until yesterday evening, we hadn't really spoken in weeks, but after one of those awkward social scrapes—I'd been window-shopping when her reflection loomed into view—we'd agreed to meet for an early drink. She chose the venue: a souped-up old boozer, its interior newly whitewashed, cruelly lit and furnished with trestle tables and school chairs—the kind you expect to find chewing gum stuck beneath, with perhaps a City Hall–style heart scratched on the back. It didn't go well. And it definitely didn't help that I told her I should have turned down the role of bridesmaid. As I'd suspected, the assignment did not end with the wedding; that was merely the seal on a contract that would have me playing bridesmaid forever. How much better if I'd simply stayed in my station as friend! But I could understand how she felt—she was living in a foreign country, clutching at nascent affinities and fellowships that might otherwise have been fleeting.

Victoria fixed me with a wobbly stare while batting off a man with a pint who was hoping to claim the spare seat beside her. "I don't have friends, I only have best friends," she declared. When had I last heard that? Suddenly the school furniture seemed maddeningly appropriate. Then the tears began to flow, and I found myself floating somewhere above it all, looking in on a scenario that must have appeared awfully like a breakup to anyone who happened to glance our way. It struck me that this makeshift, relatively new friendship was hitting the buffers with far greater resolution than any of my more intimate relationships had recently been granted. I've been broken up with often, but rarely was there a definitive bust-up like this. Phone calls would dwindle and then go unreturned. Suddenly a month would have passed and there we'd be, accidentally bumping into each other, uncertain of what kind of greeting to offer.

Wandering out into the night, I gulped the cool air. Halloween felt close and I was a witch abroad. I'd waited for her husband to come to the rescue, but still, I'd left a friend in tears. My evening wasn't about to get any easier. An hour or so later, I was edging into a birthday party filled with the married. There were no children in tow, but an improbable number of women were visibly, gloriously pregnant. I'm still in the first trimester of my chaste challenge, yet I bet they've had sex more recently. Exiling myself to a sofa in a far corner, I was joined by the only other unattached woman in the room. Actually, she was newly divorced—did that make her more or less alarming than me? Either way, there we were, two scarlet women on a beige couch.

I couldn't quite shake that witch from my mind. After all, what kinds of women were cast as witches? Lone women. Women who refused to become wives and mothers, women determined to live singly, self-sufficiently and—when not consorting with demons, presumably—chastely. It reminded me of an e-card that has been doing the rounds, in which a svelte woman with bobbed hair stands before an open wardrobe, pondering. This is her dilemma: "I can't decide this Halloween whether to go as a slutty witch, a slutty nurse, a slutty schoolgirl or just a total slut." You laugh and then you don't laugh. There's something about hearing the word *slutty* three, almost four, times over. Doesn't saying a word thrice turn it into a spell? And didn't *nun* used to be an additional jokey option? When did she vanish?

Like witch—and sex-starved minx, her more recent incarnation—nun is another traditional role for the female subversive, a way for society to contain and rationalize the loose-cannon threat she poses. Just as the Church defined *sex* for centuries (in the Dark Ages, it even reserved the right to punish husbands for glimpsing their wives naked, and wives for administering aphrodisiacs to those same peeping husbands), so it has played a major role in shaping our concept of chastity. While the sexual revolution booted the Church from the bedroom, at least in the Protestant West, we still tend to see chastity as something cloistered and removed from the world, when in fact female chastity in particular has an almost racy history.

If you were looking for chaste calendar girls, you might consider Margery Kempe, who tells her own story in one of the English language's earliest autobiographies. Born in Norfolk toward the end of the fourteenth century, she bore fourteen children before a vision persuaded her to negotiate a chaste marriage with her doting husband. She tried her hand at running a brewery and a grain mill, and journeyed as far afield as Prussia and Norway, in between finding time to antagonize the Church, which tried to ban women from preaching.

Others, too, have used chastity to challenge the confines of gender roles. In the fourth century, a woman named Ecdicia cajoled her husband into a joint vow of chastity. He promptly lapsed and took a mistress, but in renouncing the so-called "marriage debt" and reclaiming her body, Ecdicia felt entitled to cast off wifely obedience, too, and without consulting him made a large donation to a pair of wandering monks.

Even within the Church, nuns assumed roles very different from the sandal-flapping frumps of latter-day caricature. For Milton, the nun was all woman—or as much woman as he could handle, at any rate. Listen to how he calls out to "the rapt soul" in "Il Penseroso": "Come pensive nun, devout and pure,/Sober, steadfast, and demure,/All in a robe of darkest grain,/Flowing with majestic train,/ And sable stole of cypress lawn/Over thy decent shoulders drawn." Chaste, yes, but undeniably sensual, too.

Real-life nuns weren't strangers to sensuality, either. In sixteenth-century Venice, for instance, a surfeit of well-born daughters coupled with empty dowry coffers and a dearth of eligible bachelors forced many into Holy Orders. Behind tall walls, they became virtual courtesans, famed for their parties, fine clothing and high-heeled clogs.

If for some women convent life represented either prison or vocation, for others it was sanctuary. Not all who entered were virgins—some were widows, others former prostitutes. For such women, a life of chastity offered, both literally and metaphorically, a room of their own, away from the terrors of childbirth and the tedium of domestic drudgery. And while that room might seem austere, it was also furnished with luxuries like quietude and the chance to pursue educational opportunities unavailable to women in the secular world.

All this was hubble-bubbling away in my head when along came
the man I should have married, the Nice Jewish Accountant who'd
make such a perfect husband, every mother in the world must want
him for her son-in-law. It's not quite true that I should have married
him. At least I don't think he's the one cosmically destined for me. I
can't think that—it would be too gloomy, especially because, like
the rest of the room, he is very much married these days. Better to
say that he and I were best friends, a remembrance that strikes me
forcibly with my ex-friend Victoria's words still reverberating.

His was a wedding I did not go to. His fiancée sensed a history,
and though she called to invite me at the very last minute, his voice
feeding her lines in the background, I couldn't do it. I thought I
could—I got as far as dressing up and calling a cab—but once stuck
in traffic, knowing I'd be late and that even arriving on time would
not permit me a place in his life now that it had become theirs, I
paid off the driver and slipped out.

We run into each other maybe once a year now, and it's always
the same—as if no time has passed. For two years or so—those
important early-twentysomething years, full of firsts—I told him
every detail of my life and learned about his. He is religious, so to
have embarked on a physical relationship would have been tanta-
mount to an engagement, and that, in turn, would have required me
to make significant changes to my lifestyle. Was I in love with him?
I thought I was—and I was convinced enough to stay faithful to the
thought for the duration of our intense friendship. But at twenty-
three, twenty-four, I wasn't ready to get married, and eventually we
drifted apart on the tides of other, more conventional relationships.
I've since sought that same sense of spiritual and intellectual oneness from the men with whom I attained it physically. A couple of
times I've thought I found it, but it remains elusive.

. . .

Back in my accidental yoga class, our teacher is still trying to coax us into headstands. Finally I give up any pretense of participation and, flat out and breathless on my back, give in to a wave of sorrow for what has been lost. Victoria was right to have expected that making me her bridesmaid meant something. A friendship is a contract in the way that we tacitly understand all human bonds to be. Only sex seems to have become the exception. It is rogue, deregulated territory. It's cowboy country.

When the sexual revolution swept aside guilt and ignorance and repression, it also stripped away centuries of efforts to civilize sex, or at least to create a safe haven from which to explore its wilder reaches. Coasting in on post–World War II dreams of mutuality and sexual harmony, the revolution replaced outmoded marriage with chummy camaraderie. That was the ideal, anyway. The reality, for many women, was a highly partial kind of equality. When their counterculturalist unions produced offspring, they invariably found themselves stuck at home just like their mothers before them, while their partners were off furthering careers and helping other eager young women explore their sexual freedom.

Their disappointment would first rejuvenate and then derail the feminist movement, sending it careening off into outlandish, separatist extremes, as epitomized by calls for women to abort male fetuses. Along the way, the likes of Deborah Gregory would argue that women should further their quest for equality by holding themselves apart from all their relationships and striving for "emotional celibacy." By being, in other words, more masculine about it all.

Physical celibacy has intense emotional rewards. My own new-found clarity is enabling me to see that in my headlong pursuit of

sex as a route to intimacy, I've neglected gentler refrains like friendship. Into the space that sex filled, a quietness is flowing—a quietness that hasn't shut out entirely those flirty overtures of lust and
longing, but which is enabling me to pick up on subtler notes. The
next morning, yoga has left me aching in places that already feel a
little remote.

FIVE

November OR *At the Movies*

Seduction is always more singular and sublime
than sex and it commands the higher price.

—Jean Baudrillard, semiotician

I n a darkened room, the couple in front of me is tearing at each
other's clothes, their breathing ragged, their movements urgent.
Their attraction has been hand-shakingly, knee-tremblingly manifest from the moment they set eyes on each other, and as I watch
them thrust toward blissed-out oblivion, I'm feeling uncomfortably
gripped—as uncomfortably gripped as the other cinemagoers. Or
maybe more so, because beside me sits a man I once fell for with
similarly flooring, if less visually stimulating, velocity. Images from
our shared scenes stir in response to the images on-screen, and neither set is something I should be looking at if I'm to preserve my
sanity as well as my chastity.

Our liaison lasted a stormy few months and began with a simple
question: "Can I kiss you?" No one had ever asked me that before. I
was working partly as an art critic at the time, and the setting was

the private viewing of an exhibition. He was a sculptor who had interesting opinions on everything from current affairs to Turkish
coffee, and I was happy to find him there among the usual Hoxton
trendies.

The Pasha is how I've since come to think of him, partly because
in spite of having to supplement hard-earned commissions with luck
and goodwill, he cloaks himself in an aura of lazy opulence. His looks
are conventional, but he has a sculptor's appealing hands and is one
of those men who genuinely like women. Whether as cause or effect,
other men are wary of him—not that he seems to mind, and why
would he? Ordinarily, he is ringed by a harem of striking twenty-
somethings.

That evening he was on his own, and chatting, we drifted to the
fringes of the stragglers, gravitating to a small room where a projector looped dislocated images of urban something-or-other. With
that question—"Can I kiss you?"—I felt like its beam had swiveled
round on to me. I'm used to the heartbeat instant when you know
you're about to be kissed—that split second when everything seems
to freeze and then, before you've had a chance to take a preplunge
breath and fill your lungs for the torrid moments ahead, you're both
cruising in to land, eyes closed yet miraculously managing, usually,
to avoid knocking heads or noses or teeth, as if your bodies have already mapped each other's contours. This was different—it seemed
to belong to another era.

That I've forgotten my precise response is symptomatic of how
things ended between us, but I must have assented, because the next
thing I knew, the kiss had been claimed. We were sitting facing each
other on chairs and leaned into it hands free, a parody of those
sickly greetings cards in which towheaded infants pucker up for
each other. It was quite chaste, really, if you ignored the tongues.

And though it would never have occurred to me to think of the Pasha as a kissing partner, it was unexpectedly delicious.

We were among the very last to leave, and because we were both going the same way, we decided to share a cab. "I can drop you," I offered—he lived just five minutes from the gallery, against my half hour. He threw me an amused look. "You're not really going home, are you?"

There was little sign of his work in his flat—a charcoal nude abandoned on a chair, a block of plasticine molded into abstraction. The living room was sparsely furnished with an old sofa, a crimson rug and a coffee table that was really a cardboard box with an ethnic cloth thrown over it. But turning, I found that an entire wall was filled with books, extravagant not only in number but in content, too, their gilded spines revealing a great quantity of poetry, much of it translated from ornate languages.

Did I sleep with him? Well, I followed him through to the bedroom, where a mattress lay on the floor, and upon that mattress we slept, side by side. He lent me a freshly laundered Brooks Brothers dress shirt whose tails reached modestly down to my knees, the cuffs dangling so far beyond my wrists that I felt as if I'd been swigging from Alice's "Drink Me" bottle rather than cheap champagne. And the next morning—the next morning he turned to me and we melted into each other, still sleepy-slow from our late night.

Afterward, he made a pot of coffee and read me poems too sweet-seeming for the hour—like baklava for breakfast. "The soul goes dancing through the king's doorway. / Anemones blush because they have seen / the rose naked."

Romantic, except that I still had to complete my interrupted journey home from the night before—a walk of shame, only I wasn't on foot but on a bus, surrounded by commuters whose bright eyes were unsmudged by the telltale signs of yesterday evening's mascara. (There apparently exists a New York lothario who stocks his bathroom cabinet with women's potions and lotions, and I've always thought that his conquests' gratitude must eventually outweigh their dismay at having been such a foreseeable notch on his bedpost.) As I went, I registered the usual pangs of anxiety, which not even the sated feeling that follows sex after a while without can keep at bay: What had just happened? Would he call me?

Though I'm still too close to the start of my chaste year for my vow to make much of a difference—it hasn't yet tested me, nor I it—I'm surprised to find that already my perspective has altered. It's as if I'm standing off to the side slightly, even in memories. Here in the cinema, for instance, thinking about how I felt that years-ago morning, I'm struck by the fact that it didn't occur to me that *I* might be the one to call *him*. It never did. As women, we may ask a man out, split the bill, make the first move. What we can't do, decrees some unwritten, still-standing law, is be the first to call afterward. That would seem desperate, and we'd far rather feel desperate than look it.

While I was busy not calling the Pasha, he called me. A couple of days later, we met up. On one level I knew that we had no future together—his life was in flux, and he was in no position to commit, which was what I wanted, even if I didn't acknowledge it. Moreover, I feared that his heart belonged to a girl who'd gone before me, the one whose photograph still sat on a table in a shadowy corner of his flat. Nevertheless, for a few months I was so completely under his spell that I refused to see it.

That spell was sex, yet it's largely in terms of food that I recall the relationship. It coincided with my giving up almost two decades of vegetarianism. I remember leaving his flat one Saturday morning to go shopping with one or two members of The Group. Removed from his presence, I suddenly realized how famished I was. I dived into a deli for a sandwich, which I ate as I strolled through lunchtime crowds toward Oxford Street. It was tuna salad, and my first bite in twenty years brought back taste memories that I hadn't known existed. Another time, sitting on the Pasha's saggy couch, I twirled spaghetti Bolognese round my fork and reacquainted myself with red meat. That these newly released memories dated from childhood gave them a cosseting coziness—feelings that became tangled up with my feelings for the man sitting beside me, watching. Of course, there were a few more adult foods that I'd never tasted. Caviar was one of them, and it was the Pasha who fed me my first spoonful.

It proved hard to kick, the vegetarianism, and you might wonder why I was even trying. At age eight, my principles had been determined by the calves and lambs that I used to pass on the way to school, but by the time I met the Pasha, my dietary preference had become simple habit. Others didn't see it that way—to them, it was an intrinsic part of who I was. More specifically, men saw me as a vegetarian girl, and while I wasn't entirely sure what that meant, I sensed a link in their minds between a woman's appetite for rare steak and her sexual appetite. A vegetarian girl was drippy, passive—which was ironic, because it could be said that passivity was what first led me into the Pasha's arms. His questioning—his "Can I kiss you?"—had flustered me. I'd always liked to think of romance as being more predestined than that.

In the years since, we've become firm friends, thanks mainly to his persistence. Back when we broke up—on my birthday, no less—I felt like he'd maneuvered me into it, casting me as the villain when I was an equal victim. For six months afterward, I tried not speaking to him. Eventually I realized that I enjoyed having the occasional drink with him, and chatting now and then on the phone. Though our friendship is strictly platonic, I know that, like those carnivorous taste memories, the memory of the carnal knowledge we shared is preserved somewhere. It's shaded with entitlement, as if we'll always own a little of each other, which perhaps we shall. We move on, but years and relationships later, given the right combination of time and place, a look or a word can spring the lock behind which we've stowed those memories. Multisensory experiences—they are the emotional equivalent of a peep show.

For me, it's Jake's smile and the Pasha's hands—those same hands that I've watched spoon foie gras onto toast and caress my nipple. Unexpectedly alone with each other or merely thrown out of context, such attributes will sweep us back. In a world that casts us as consumers in every aspect of our lives, we're primed to crave novelty, but sometimes it is what Philip Roth's Zuckerman refers to in *Exit Ghost* as "The emotional boomerang of erotic attachment" that slays us. If untested potential captures our romantic imaginations, it's the forgotten familiar that fires our carnal fancies.

And yet those supposedly personal images, where do they really come from? We're still sitting side by side in the cinema, the Pasha and I, watching actors act out great sex in a mediocre film. Thanks to closed-set scenes, we all have a highly defined notion of how sex looks—or how it looks in the movies, at any rate. For how it looks in real life, there are documentaries like *A Girl's Guide to 21st Century Sex,* which thoughtfully deployed a tiny internal camera to show us sex from the vagina's viewpoint.

At the steamier, seamier end of the spectrum, recent surveys highlight teenagers as one of porn's biggest consumer groups, and they're tuning in, they say, partly to pick up tips on technique. But what we don't really gain from visual exposure to sex, however explicit, is a sense of how it feels. As in all spheres of life, we know more, yet what we know from direct experience is diminishing. Much of what we do learn we don't fully internalize, either—we don't need to, with the Internet functioning as a kind of giant communal exomemory. When it comes to sex, we learn less and less from hands-on trial and error, from fooling around, and more from sitting around watching what appears to feel good to other people.

On-screen, it sometimes seems as if even the characters themselves are experiencing the situation from without. In Cynthia Mort's HBO drama *Tell Me You Love Me* (2007), the sex was X-rated and bleakly unerotic. Shot entirely on Super 16, the series captured intimacy from unexpected angles and at clinically close range. There was full-frontal male nudity and little makeup or music to mask what was going on. Frequently the camera caught something less gynecological but more revealing: the eyes of a character looking anywhere but at his or her partner, disconnected from the moment, pursuing some private hurt or grievance that not even the most intense physical contact could touch. They were stripped naked but still fully clothed in their neuroses.

Mostly, staged sex seems to be pretty hot sex—studios hire sex choreographers to make sure of it. It's hardly surprising, then, that American researchers have found that teenagers who think telly portrays sex accurately are far more likely to be dissatisfied with their first real experience of intercourse. Climax proves anticlimactic. Though we're all trained to want sex, the "sex" we're sold on is a hybrid that bears scanty resemblance to sex as most of us experience it, at least to start with.

And where does this leave privacy? Aside from the odd documentary, we know that what we're observing is fiction, which is why our protests focus on CCTV rather than dolly-mounted cameras, and yet every time the director beckons us into the bedroom, our own imaginary spaces are being invaded. All the way back in 1970, novelist J. G. Ballard told a *Penthouse* interviewer that "organic sex, body against body, skin area against skin area, is becoming no longer possible, simply because if anything is to have any meaning for us it must take place in terms of the values and experiences of the media landscape." Advances in technology and communication were among the things that he said were "beginning to reach into our lives and change the interior design of our sexual fantasies." Almost forty years on, that design scheme has become bordello kitsch. If it's titillating, it's also isolating. We're kept outside the experience—we're passive. Online porn and neighborhood lap-dancing clubs do more of the same—they cast the viewers as voyeurs, isolating them from their own desire.

The seventeenth-century memoirist François de la Rochefoucauld maintained that people would never fall in love if they had not heard love talked about. We're arguably still more receptive to visual narratives.

Propped beside my bed is a postcard. Titled "Four Scenes of Courtship," it shows the carved ivory cover of a wax writing tablet from fourteenth-century France, which now resides in the Metropolitan Museum of Art. Arranged two up, two down, and each framed by an archway, this quartet of scenes reads like a storyboard.

In the first scene, a man pursues a woman who flaps demurely in a parody of rejection. His hand appears to hover over her breast, though depth of field is tricky to gauge. The second scene shows them sitting side by side. A pet fox is on her lap, looking up at her. The man balances his ankle jauntily on his knee, and his arm snakes around her back. With his free hand, he cups her chin. He's obviously a fast worker, because come the third image, they are playing board games together. Chess, it looks like, and their gestures speak of some kind of spat. Has he been cheating? Has she? By the fourth, he has clinched the deal: kneeling before her while she stands, her arm resting on his shoulder, his on her belly. Either she is pregnant or he is proposing.

There is something cheering about such step-by-step simplicity, enlivened as it is by pursuit and tenderness and companionship, all easily legible despite the players' age-soiled features. Most irresistible is the second panel: that gentle cupping of her chin, the caress that probably began on her cheek and slid suggestively down. Letting someone touch your face like that—it's about as intimate and loving as it gets.

Despite the impudent ambiguity of that hand-on-breast opener (should it seem so odd that while our sexual inhibitions have relaxed, our sense of personal space has become more sharply honed?), if this really were a storyboard it would carry a PG certificate, and yet it connotes far greater intimacy than most of today's sex scenes.

The infamous Hays Production Code, enforced in Hollywood from 1934 until 1968, banned the depiction of everything from safecracking to childbirth, but it saved its most rigorous rules for the representation of sex. Nudity, adultery and "excessive and lustful kissing" all became outlawed activities the moment the director yelled, "Action!"

Is it significant that Hollywood's golden age coincided with this period of censorship? It wasn't merely what audiences saw and heard that was censored—even symbolism was kept chaste. Or it was supposed to be. Maybe my vow has made me extrasensitized, but watching some of those Hays-era films for the first time—really watching them as an adult, rather than as a child, when I was aware only of their black-and-whiteness, their incredible wordiness—I'm surprised by how smoldering they are. Because physical gratification risked blue-penciling, it was delayed and delayed and delayed. Men and women circle the unmentionable together through charged badinage that draws them ever closer, sparring with lines so nimble that they seem not merely scripted but choreographed. There is nothing that chaste eyes may not see, but the effects are sizzling.

More striking still is the caliber of roles written for female leads. Take George Cukor's *Adam's Rib*. Released in 1949, it seems, superficially, every bit as dated as its age suggests. Katharine Hepburn plays Amanda Bonner, a lawyer who invokes feminist rhetoric in her defense of a woman who has pulled a gun on her philandering husband. Across the court is the prosecuting counsel, Amanda's own husband, Adam, played by Spencer Tracy. As the case gathers pace, it makes the headlines and puts the Bonners' marriage under massive and hugely entertaining strain. The arguments voiced in court by day follow them home, where they're put to the test each evening as they entertain dinner guests or indulge in an almost risqué massage scene. After much yelling and door slamming, Adam storms out.

Part of the film's appeal is that famous Spence-Kate chemistry, but it's also the script. Written by Ruth Gordon and Garson Kanin, another husband-and-wife team, it casts husband and wife as equals and gives Hepburn some of the sharpest, wittiest lines of her career. There she is in 1949, fighting for equality in the public sphere. Contrast her role with, say, Jennifer Aniston's Brooke in *The Break-Up*, Peyton Reed's 2006 romantic comedy. Almost sixty years and all that social change later, and she is fighting for a far less evolved kind of equality, without getting any of the good lines, either. She wants to make her ex, Vince Vaughn's Gary, grow up and treat her like a human being, which, in terms of the script, makes her an almighty drag. There is no sex and little love, and at the peak of the film's dramatic arc, Brooke is battling merely to be seen by Gary.

As veteran feminist Betty Friedan complained to *People* magazine, "We need to see men and women as equal partners, but it's hard to think of movies that do that. When I talk to people, they think of movies of 45 years ago! Hepburn and Tracy!" A further decade has passed since she said that, but things have hardly improved. It can't be this simple—women couldn't have lost their voices when they gave up their on-screen chastity. But never mind equality— how much more fun Kate and company seem! They are carefree and smart, blessed with style and attitude. They often deliver the punch lines, too, unlike Kathleen Kelly, the blustering heroine played by Meg Ryan in the contemporary classic *You've Got Mail,* itself a remake of the 1940 hit *The Shop Around the Corner.* Though I love Ryan's film, it is, as academic Maria DiBattista observes in *Fast-Talking Dames,* about a woman who can never find the right words at the right moment, and when she finally does, she regrets it.

But back to the sex, because I admit that in this, my third month, I am beginning to feel its lack. Received wisdom says that it was the Hays Code that first divorced sex from love in the cinema, partnering it instead with that other outlawed emotion, violence. Freed from Hays, Hollywood gloried in shiny, sweaty, pumped-up sex. Sex with sixties soundtracks, seventies hairdos and eighties fake tans. Some of it was indeed violent but much was loving—in fact it was the easiest way to show love: simply cut to tangled satin sheets and flashes of flesh.

Lately, however, love and sex really do seem to have split up. Now that every kind of sex has been shown on camera—even intercourse that was for real, rather than simulated—directors seem to have lost interest in it. Today, love is the hot topic. Yes, masturbation is big in indie movies right now (Noah Baumbach even got Nicole Kidman's character to do it in 2007's *Margot at the Wedding*), but mightn't that just be a metaphor for sexual alienation? And while full-frontal male nudity remains voguish—Bart Simpson has bared all, and producer-director Judd Apatow has publicly vowed to include a penis in every film he makes—those penises don't see much action. In *Superbad,* also released in 2007, the teen protagonists end up deferring sex and forging romantic friendships instead. In *Knocked Up,* released that same summer, Seth Rogen's sad, ultimately sweet slacker (whose life's work is, incidentally, a movie database of female nudity) gets insanely lucky when he beds Katherine Heigl's blond, up-and-coming telly presenter, and immediately his fun is over. He may be too drunk to remember anything about it, but he's got her pregnant.

And then there's Craig Gillespie's *Lars and the Real Girl.* Premiered in the autumn of 2007, its title character logs on to find himself a girl. When she comes to visit, she travels DHL and arrives on his doorstep in a large crate. She is a life-size, anatomically correct "love doll," yet over the coming weeks, she and Lars sleep in separate rooms and share only one on-screen kiss, going against all that you'd expect from a film about a twenty-seven-year-old virgin loner whose fly is frequently undone and his mail-order sex doll. It becomes, in short, a love story. (Of course it doesn't bode at all well for actresses that a female lead goes to what one character terms "a big plastic thing.")

The same is true on the small screen. When HBO aired *Tell Me You Love Me,* ABC countered with *Pushing Daisies,* in which the hero has found his heroine but cannot so much as shake her hand, be-cause any bodily contact with him will kill her outright.

Compared with those earlier black-and-white dalliances, today's on-screen romances can seem—well, chaste.

. . .

Hays-era filmmakers were arbiters of delayed gratification. Once a necessity, it's become a near impossibility. Relationships move so swiftly to the bedroom that there is no courtship storyboard, but I've glimpsed it accidentally with the Beau. Geography, coupled with a disconcerting age gap, has made our pace dawdling, and yet looking back on our unconsummated times together, they are the closest I've experienced to romance in a very long time.

Early on, after what was maybe our second or third dinner date, we strolled toward the tube together. It was autumn, and mist swirled around the streetlamps poetically, drawing out the mulchy scent of bright leaves trampled underfoot. As we passed a bulky red-brick building set back from the road, a big band struck up within. Following its sound, we found ourselves in a dance hall filled with men and women in fifties clothing, jiving athletically—and yes, sexily. It was as if we'd parted the night and stepped back in time. Returning to our own age, we ended up sitting in the rafters of a jazz bar. The Beau fingered a bracelet that dangled from my wrist and tried to persuade me to dance. We didn't in the end, not that night, but the rhythm of those big-skirted, spivvy-suited jivers pulsed through the rest of our evening.

My sole experience of dancing lessons was in New York, as part of my bridesmaid's preparation for Victoria's wedding. We women had only to follow, but it turned out we were incapable of being led. In exasperation, our teacher—an ethereally skinny young man—threatened to employ blindfolds. There was also the question of embarrassment. Our partners were the groomsmen—men we knew, at least a little. Yet finding ourselves holding and being held in such ritualized positions, we blushed. Eye contact made us squirm. Our palms grew as clammy as those of fifties sweethearts.

It was somehow sexy, but in a new, foreign way that we didn't know how to deal with.

There are other things as sexy as sex, too. I learned this when I was fourteen and a new boy named Luke joined my class. He was fair-haired and smart enough, but quietly so, cool though inconspicuously—his father was in the forces and he knew the drill when it came to starting over. Like me, he played the clarinet, and that he did with winning disregard for the high-school rubric of blending in and keeping your head down. He did it brilliantly, and he didn't care what people made of it.

Luke and I began sharing lessons. We started playing duets— jazz duets, full of the sensual drag and wanton lilt of syncopation. The tunes we learned evoked smoky dive bars and early-hours abandon, or else wartime dance floors given a defiant edge by death's close-hovering presence. We knew nothing of any of it, of course, but occasionally a sashaying phrase would bring us within brushing distance.

We spent our lunch hours in the music room, whose windows looked directly out onto the sports field, giving us a glimpse of our opposites—the runners and jumpers, the shouters. Yet indoors we shared secrets that they, in all their lithe, outdoors physicality, would never have guessed at.

I've a particularly vivid memory in which Luke and I are standing side by side, close enough to read from a single sheet of music. It's summer and we're both in regulation thin white shirts, our sleeves rolled up. But more thrilling is the musical closeness. The rhythmic push and pull of our entwined melodies describes something I knew only through music back then. Even now, it's hard to think of a sensation to match it. It is, I suppose, sex. Sunlight pools on the page and exams must be near because I'm acutely aware of this moment as a passing moment. Even from within, it is tinged with nostalgia.

I'll remember this as a kind of idyll, I think to myself. And I do, though an idyll of something I've come to understand only years later.

While most of us can tell the story of our first time, we lose sight of that other first—the first time we really grasped the mechanics of sex. I can't remember how old I was, but my mother assures me that when the time came to explain the logistics, I flatly refused to believe her. It all seemed so outlandish. I preferred my own version, in which a tadpolelike sperm somehow wriggled across the bedclothes from Daddy to Mummy.

I promptly forgot about it until puberty beckoned, and sex then became something else—a feeling. Maybe that's how we all first experience it—a flush made hotter for being illicit, occasioned by stumbling across the naughty bits in a book, for instance. For me, this happened when I was about eleven. We were on holiday and staying in a converted Welsh chapel, of all places. The rain that had kept us indoors was drumming on a skylight as I roamed the bookshelves, and there it was—a book full of naughty bits. Probably just *The Joy of Sex,* it now occurs to me. There were images, but they were not like a movie—they were the kind of soft pencil outlines that your mind could color in.

As we grow older, sex comes to seem like the answer to other mysteries that call out from childhood. It's an answer—a retort, at least—to death, the darkest of them all. And for a long time, it seemed to me that it was the response to a kind of yearning I'd been feeling since before I even had a word for it. If I had to conjure up

a single memory to encapsulate it, it would be this: I'm seven—
or eight, or maybe six—and I can't sleep. The sheets are tucked tight
around me and a story-time hush hovers in my pink-papered room,
whose walls are alive with tiny butterflies. I picked out this paper
myself—the curtains as well, which depict a big top, its bright
bunting framing jugglers, seals and trapezes flying through a star-
spangled blank.

The house is an old house, and it sighs and creaks at will. A
thatched roof adds a musty note to the scent that means home to
me—wood, wool, things from outdoors brought in. From downstairs
I can hear the radio, or is it the television? A laugh, perhaps, either
canned or real, and later, the abrupt clang of cutlery on crockery—a
jangling discontent that occasionally erupts in shouting and
slammed doors.

All of this is the background noise to my childhood—noise I
would hear only were it to be silenced. What's keeping me awake is
something else. It's inspired by the season, the hour, the light: early
summer, early evening, sunset peach. Even now, the call of a pi-
geon—that sort of melodious throat clearing—will take me right
back there, to that low-ceilinged house whose squat windows looked
out onto a green, tree-filled garden just big enough to suggest vistas,
possibility, a beyond that was being kept from me.

I can now see that the answer to that feeling was not sex—at
least, not of the hasty, low-commitment kind. I suppose music had
seemed an answer at one point, but sex—especially as played out on
the big screen—is such a potent idea that music fell by the wayside.
Sexologist Henry Havelock Ellis—in his personal life, one of the
kinky characters sometimes drawn to the field—wrote in his essay
collection *On Life and Sex* that "the sexual embrace can only be compared with music and with prayer." That same embrace—or a

pumped-up, airbrushed version of it—has since replaced religious devotion. In a recent blog post for the *New York Times,* Sari Locker wrote of "the oozing exploitation of sex on television, movies, magazines, books, and the internet," declaring us to be living through "The Era of Sexual Pressure." Locker is an academic and the author of a somewhat less than academic volume, *The Complete Idiot's Guide to Amazing Sex.* "In all my years as a sex educator," she continues, "I've never seen such a huge gap between the reality of ordinary people's sex lives and the myths about sex from pop culture that they're taking to heart." Yet even as they raise our expectations of sex, those images shrink down its definition, narrowing our erotic vocabulary and denying us the chance to conjure up our own fantasies, to make sex the form of self-expression that it should, in part, be.

Delayed gratification doesn't just mean that the climax, when it finally does arrive, is bigger and better, but, as all those black-and-white movies show, it makes the world sexier and the sex itself more multidimensional. Or is that my vow speaking? In which case, I've just proven the last bit, so there's hope for the first.

SIX

December OR Party Time

Lechery, lechery; still, wars and lechery:
nothing else holds fashion.

—Shakespeare, *Troilus and Cressida*

There is a man standing on my doorstep and he's carrying the most all-out gorgeous bouquet I've ever seen. Muffled against the cold, smiling quizzically—probably wondering if there's any hope I'll stop eyeballing the flowers long enough to let him in—he holds them out to me. Even in the sparse glow of the hallway light spilling over my shoulders, they are redder than red. Red tulip petals cupping sooty hearts; tightly clenched red peonies—or something closely related to a peony; and, of course, red roses, some just buds, others already opening up with abandon. Rapt, I feel their color tinge my cheeks. When did I last blush?

If I were the swooning type, I would already have sunk to the floor in coils. After just three chaste months, I may well have become that type, but there isn't the space to crumple elegantly in my hallway, and I fancy it takes practice to achieve without injury, so instead I step aside and let my dinner guest enter. Together we do a funny little dance, attempting a kiss on the cheek or a friendly hug or even a handshake around these magnificent blooms. They fill the space between us, growing bigger and redder by the second, muffling the sound of a half dozen hungry friends gathered in the living room.

Flowers are my biggest weakness. I've never aspired to a garden, and pot plants tend to wither in my care, but cut flowers seem magical, whether they're half-price tulips or heavy-headed lilies. I could suggest that it has to do with the way they combine vivacity with mortality—plucked in their prime, they put everything into those brief-lived bursts of color and scent—but really it's nothing so ponderous. They are frivolous, they are essential—it's as simple as that.

Oddly, they don't have much to do with romance in my mind, either. In my family, we women either buy our own or receive them from one another. I don't recall my father ever presenting my mother with flowers when I was growing up. Every Friday morning she'd bicycle to the nearest town—a two-street town barely more than a village—for the Women's Institute market. It was held in a community hall that smelled of dust and age, and there she'd vie with a local painter for the boldest and brightest, returning with Michaelmas daisies, lupines, foxgloves and homemade lemon sponge slices.

Her relationship with her own mother was complicated—far more complicated than I could have known as a child, though even then I grasped something of its wonky dimensions. Because she wanted her daughters to have a grandmother, there was a visit every few months. Granny had a black Lab named Bessie—a clumsy, keen mutt who was overweight enough for it to hurt when she trod on our sandaled toes, and who loved nothing more than having her coat vacuumed. As we sat at the table, swinging our legs and dunking white bread in our boiled eggs, she'd sit underneath it, her tail thunking on the linoleum in anticipation of crumbs. Afterward, we'd visit Nettie, the goat who lived among the hens but frequently escaped to graze off the roses. Before we left, our grandmother would give my sister and me a bag of candy each and pick a bunch of flowers from the garden for our mum, wrapping them in wet newspaper so they'd survive the train journey back.

When it was Granny's turn to visit us, I'd sit in the living-room window, watching for her arrival. Behind me all my favorite dolls would be lined up for her to inspect. When she finally stepped through the door, she'd glance vaguely in their direction before wandering out with a cup of tea to the shed, from which my father ran a picture-framing business. She was a man's woman, it seems to me now, not a little girl's, and definitely not a doll's. We'd all troop down to the village for cake, and when eventually Granny left, she'd be clutching a posy picked from our garden. In each instance the flowers seemed meaningful—nothing as definitive as a peace offering, but something similar.

Until this evening, I'd just twice been given flowers by men. The boy I most wanted to come to my twentieth birthday party sent a bouquet instead of himself, and Dan gave me freesias and daffs one Valentine's Day. Yet now, a season into my year of chastity, here is a man clutching this outrageously lovely bunch, a bunch that far exceeds the duty of a guest at a last-minute supper party.

Mr. Vermilion is how he becomes fixed in my mind from this point on. The name fits him in other ways, too, with its echoed riches. He is an architect and looks the part: auburn curls, elegantly cut suit, a brightly striped scarf that he's unwinding from his neck. There is something slightly out of time about his appearance—despite the splashy scarf, his suaveness has a sepia quality to it. His voice is deep and treacly, oozing merriment. He laughs a lot and his laugh enlivens his face with gentle comedy, making him less Cary Grant, more Jack Lemmon.

With the festive season getting under way, Mr. Vermilion's bouquet is a reminder of a more ancient kind of pageantry—of evergreens and mistletoe and pagan feasting. It also whispers of the language of flowers, which is just as racy in its way as lacy stockings and smoky eye makeup. These natural titillations even come with their own antidote—*Vitex agnus-castus,* otherwise known as the chaste tree due to its small, round, pepperlike fruits, which were used by monks to dampen the libido.

Freud, we're told, made the whole world sexy. "Analyse any human emotion, no matter how far it may be removed from the sphere of sex, and you are sure to discover somewhere the primal impulse to which life owes its perpetuation," he lectured. The same went for dreams, most of which he interpreted as expressions of sexual desire. His list of sex-related dream symbols ran from the obvious (sticks, tree trunks, umbrellas) to the kinkily bizarre (smooth walls and tables set for dinner), in between encompassing everything from complicated machinery to cravats and nail files. As a post-Freudian society, we might also add abstracts like childhood and friendship.

These lists are near-poetry to read, and yes, they send the chaste mind roaming in ill-advised directions. But going back to that first declaration: just how sexy can a primal impulse be? Mightn't it be that at the same time as expanding our inventory of sex-related *objets* to include staircases and stoves, Freud also narrowed our definition of sexiness?

As MIT philosophy professor Irving Singer writes in *The Pursuit of Love,* in attributing any interest that we humans hold for one another to reproductive energy, "[Freud] failed to appreciate the degree to which pleasures of seeing, touching, tasting, smelling, and even yearning might be sexual in another fashion." They might, Singer goes on, be erotic rather than libidinal.

I met Mr. Vermilion a few weeks ago, when I was sent to interview him.

Clutching a map, I'd picked my way through a patch of town that I knew only from the windows of buses. It was a typical London jumble of balconied council blocks and well-fortified Victorian terraces. A weathered St. George's Cross drooped outside a pub, a shop sold everything and nothing. Rounding a corner, I came upon what looked like a mini industrial estate, and it was here, apparently, that Mr. Vermilion lived.

He was younger than I'd anticipated—in his early forties, whereas my imagination had added a decade. His home was a bright white cube and felt curated rather than lived in, so it seemed surreal that it should contain anything as cozy as tea and biscuits, but that was exactly what he produced while I set about recording us, pulling out a notepad that I'd forget to glance at for the next couple of hours.

There are two distinct approaches that a journalist may take in an interview. You either play nice, in the hope that you can lull your interviewee into betraying something, something beyond the carefully constructed front being offered to you, or else you get mean—you needle and you prod and you back him into a corner, again in the hope that he'll let down his defenses. For reasons more cowardly than tactical, I favor the former strategy. Sometimes it works, and sometimes—well, sometimes you're doomed to failure whatever you do. But Mr. Vermilion, he was a series of surprises.

We sat side by side at a long table, facing French windows that gave out onto a tiny courtyard where the afternoon light was already dimming. I want to say that conversation flowed, but it didn't—it did something better. While questions were asked and answers given, it looped loquaciously, ambling unself-consciously down cul-de-sacs, taking the scenic route. More tea was made, and those biscuits were good. The paper had sent along a photographer, whose arrival ordinarily would have been my time's-up signal, but we talked on as Mr. Vermilion was maneuvered into a pose and flashes went off. The photographer was surprised that we'd only just met.

As an interviewer, you are licensed to ask all sorts of nosy questions. Ages ago, an editor called me midinterview to say that he'd just heard that the wunderkind pianist facing me, fiddling with a swizzle stick, was newly engaged to a wunderkind cellist. Could I check if it was so? A mischievous smile played on the musician's lips, though his answer was more than full: "Would you answer that question if you were me?"

In some ways, it should be the perfect way to meet and vet men— I even wound up with Mr. Vermilion's CV to help with fact-checking. Sometimes it can feel like a kind of heightened speed-dating, though the surprise should not be how much an interview can resemble a first date, but how much a first date—and a second, sometimes even a third—can resemble an interview. We are all so good at playing ourselves, and the more relationships we rack up, the better at it we become. We can even carry it off in bed.

You'd think that Christmas would be the seasonal exception, the moment when we drop the act and become ourselves. After all, it's one big exception—the time of year when everyone gives in to a kind of elemental pleasure seeking, spending more, eating more, misbehaving more. Though it shouldn't, the word *orgy* springs to mind, and I scurry to chase it out. With Baby Jesus all but swept

aside, it's hard not to feel the approach of the darkest day as the fes-
tivities gather pace.

Cast as a kind of sexual Scrooge, I'm hyperaware of my vow. I'd
always thought of Christmas as a time for letting your hair down,
but that is precisely what it isn't about, especially for women. If we
do let our hair down, it's only having first straightened it to within
an inch of its life; otherwise we pin and spray it into complex updos.
We treat our flesh with similar punitiveness, squeezing into items
that may be more technologically advanced than corsets but which
perform the exact same functions, molding, holding and generally
squishing our bodies into impossible ideals. (So much for the rational dress movement.) And then there's the makeup.

But I'll stop right there, because dressing up is fun, and as long as
there are women in the world who must court disfigurement whenever they step out of their homes wearing lipstick, it is not something to bewail. What strikes me now, though, is the extent to which
we apply personalities, too. Glossy magazines at either end of the
market are filled with tips for making ourselves more appealing to
the opposite gender. Not even the men's mags are immune. The holiday has grown so commercialized that no one really thinks to complain about it any longer, but as an outsider in all this merriment,
I'm struck not by how much we consume but by how enslaved we
are as vendors of our own charms. Sex appeal is all, and we become
so caught up in its pursuit—or manufacture, because we're encouraged to think that it can be created—we forget to question whether
this particular brand of sex appeal is something we actually want.

We feel our way toward our sexual identity, and most of our point-
ers come not from within but from without. They fill films and TV

shows, pop lyrics and the language itself. At age two and a half, I named a beloved toy giraffe Bimbo. This was the late seventies, a time before junior pole-dancing kits, pink "Lolita" beds and juvenile editions of women's magazines, like *Elle Girl*. Nor were there Bratz dolls, all pouting lips and come-hither eyes as they call out from chocolate-bar wrappers positioned just within reach of the chubby hands of stroller-riding toddlers.

What we did have were Sindys and Barbies. Even at six, we girls seemed to know that the dolls' smooth plastic physiques were communicating something to us. What exactly, we weren't quite sure, but maybe we sensed that we weren't meant to know just yet— maybe that was why we preferred to discard their tan, toned, pneumatic-busted bodies and play only with their pretty heads. Or perhaps we were just copying the big girls. At playtime, they would stand in a circle like giant cannibals, their fingers adorned with the heads of Enchanted Evening Barbie and Starlight Sindy. They'd groom them, debate hairstyles, and occasionally one of the heads would unburden her woes. Far from the glamorous lives that their creators intended, these dolls seemed to lead lives of quietly desperate drudgery. They fretted about picking the kids up on time from school, and dreamed up new flavors for the SodaStream. At the end of the school day, the coiffed heads would be reunited unblinkingly with their bodies, though there often seemed to be a spare lolling in the bottom of someone's schoolbag.

Of all the most desirable Sindy accessories, shoes topped the bill. They may have been fashioned from squishy plastic, but they had heels, and high heels, along with pointy toes and the brazen sheen of patent leather, were exactly what I yearned for in a shoe from the age of seven. Needless to say, those were not the shoes I got. What I got were round-toed buckle-ups with, if I was lucky, some punched-out detail. Every year, the back-to-school routine included a daylong tussle with my mother, trawling shops in search of compromise footwear.

We'd almost always end up in the same store, where the kids' department was hidden down in the basement. A low ceiling emphasized the eleventh-hour chaos: the stewed air, discarded boxes and stray sneakers, the banquettes where parents sat in heaps, worn out and weighed down by shopping bags spilling set squares and rulers. Often, one of the younger children would be writhing on the floor, having a full-on temper tantrum that suddenly made me look good—until the sales assistant lifted the lids off her various boxed offerings. With my foot secured in one of those special all-round measuring devices, wedged at the toe and taped in across its width, I saw red. "I am never, ever, *ever* wearing *those!*" I proclaimed, as snotty as an apprentice fashion journalist. In ugly-sister mode, the discrepancy between my brutish behavior and the princesslike footwear that I was demanding was quite lost on me.

My mum would by this point have given up trying to curb my worst excesses, given up pleading and placating, and wandered off, ostensibly to do more browsing but also in an attempt to disown the obnoxious brat who looked a lot like me. Along with all the other parents, she knew that these brown-uniformed women had a secret weapon. Once you had consented to try on a pair of shoes that your parent had consented to pay for, you were marched off to the mouth of the storeroom, where an older, sterner lady with fingers of steel would crouch down and pinch the shoe and your chubby foot with it, checking to make sure that you had room to grow and that the style matched your overall foot shape.

My feet are pretty much the only part of me that I outright like. (I'm not so keen on other people's, so it's never developed into a fetish.)

Be that as it may, they are sturdy feet. An unkind observer might almost call them square, and to the pinching witch whose job it was to deny any child a shoe she actually liked, they were a double F, and thus terminally unsuited to anything with even the hint of a taper at its toe.

When were shoes first given names? I wonder. Of all the most inappropriately named items, those shoes, the ones I ended up with year after year, have to be up there with hurricanes and flat-pack furniture. They had names like Doreen or Patricia, and it would be on the bus home, passing through streets empty with lateness, that I'd spot it stamped on top of the box, right beside their size and double-F stigma. Wrung out though I'd be from the drama of it all, that name would seem like the final ignominy. Just a name, yet always such a dowdy-seeming name, or, worse yet, the name of a girl in my class, a mean girl whose own shoes—patent and pointy—would flaunt a flashy name like Stacey or Estelle.

My friend Tracy was not a mean girl but she did have the shoes for it. She was an only child who lived in a trim close of newly built bungalows. When I played with my sister, we invented epic action dramas. With my friend Emma, we were sleuths, cracking cases that lasted days on end. But Tracy and I only ever played at being grown-ups. Our grown-ups led very dull lives, too. All we really did during these games was parade up and down the smooth new tarmac surrounding her bungalow, but we seemed to sense even at ten that being grown-up had something to do with our walk, with the way we held ourselves, with something projected from within. The only props we needed for this game were heels and handbags, and Tracy had an eye-popping collection of both. I don't think I've ever worn matching shoes and clutch bag since, but that's how we would totter along together.

One day, as we waited for my father to pick me up, she presented me with a shopping bag. Inside were the shoes I'd been wearing that afternoon. "They're yours," she told me. I clutched them tightly the whole way home, rushing directly up to my room to see how they looked, even though I'd been wearing them all afternoon. They were gray, with tiny stiletto kitten heels and those pointy toes I so longed for. On the outer edge of each were two tiny buttons, also gray. They were everything that I'd dreamed of, and yet, sitting perched on the edge of my girlish pink bed, they looked different from the shoes I'd worn in mine and Tracy's make-believe world.

I knew my mother would be appalled but couldn't have guessed that she'd make me throw them out. I fought for them, of course, but without much heart: somewhere deep down I knew she was right. Before I bade them farewell, I took one last stroll in them, hobbling round the graveled yard at the back of our house. Without the tarmac, the crisp clack-clack-clack of my heels was missing, and so, too, was that giddy sense of grown-up-ness—it was the sound that had made them.

It would be another dozen years before I owned a pair to rival those. The heels we all wore at university were innocent and clumpy (Mavis and Maud might've been their names), but a few months into my first real job, I bought a pair of slip-ons, reduced from half a week's wages to half a day's. Their kitten heels were so low they were almost flat, but they rang out thrillingly on pavements and in the glass-domed atrium that I dashed across every morning, late to my desk. Better yet, their toes were pointed, long and low-cut. "Toe cleavage" one male friend dubbed the effect, and his eyes would drop teasingly to my feet whenever he saw me in them.

I enjoyed those shoes so much that I bought an almost identical pair before the sale ended. I'd been growing out a mistaken haircut—that short-back-and-swooping-sides look worn by Victoria Beckham, as rendered by a trainee hairdresser at a discount rate—and around about then some swing and flick finally returned to it. Suddenly, men who'd never glanced at me were looking my way. Maybe it was triggered by something else altogether, but it certainly coincided with the shoes and the hair.

Sometimes, if I haven't worn them in a while, I still feel like I'm dressing up when I put on heels. I'll be running round at home, late as ever. Doing everything in the wrong order, I'll find myself only partially clothed but already in those shoes, and the extra height they'll give me will transform a task like brushing my teeth.

My Christmas party card is almost empty this year, but there is one I'm curious about, and I intend to wear heels. Its sender is N. We met at a music festival three or four years ago, and though we've not actually seen each other since (he lives in New York but has only just moved there from Austin, Texas), we've made periodic attempts to, and just when I think he's vanished from my life, up he'll pop again via e-mail. There's not much more that I can tell you about him, except that he is my age, is a rock guitarist (think session musician rather than front man) and is the only man I've yet seen almost—almost—able to carry off a ponytail. Right now, he's spending some time back in England, and the party is to be held at the riverside home of his older brother, who has done well in finance.

As it happens, the Beau is also going to be in town, and because we haven't seen each other in a while, he is staying at my place. Come party day, he arrives at my office straight from the airport, and I wander down to the lobby to meet him, experiencing that sudden jolt of seeing someone you know well thrown out of context. In that instant, I realize that we'd gotten to know each other in his world—a world in which I was invariably younger and less accomplished than anyone he introduced me to. Newly landed in my world he looks tired and seems shorter, too, in a way that isn't entirely about my heels. As we head for the escalator, I resist the urge to pluck a piece of lint from the shoulder of his jacket.

The Beau and N don't appear to hit it off. If they were women, it would be verbal, but as they're men, it's physical. Not that they're throwing punches. Instead they do that strange circling thing men do. Eventually N thrusts a plate of crudités at the Beau. The Beau proceeds to wolf down a handful of carrot sticks. Spying a plate of smoked salmon sandwiches—or is it the striking redhead?—he stalks off to a far corner, abandoning both me and his standoff with N.

N, I should confide, is rather more attractive than I remember. He's wearing a suit, which seems a pleasant gesture of respect to his big brother, and there's even a tie around his neck, though he's been yanking at it periodically—a companion gesture to the raking of his hand through his hair, a mop of wheaten curls that, happily for me, have been cut too short for a ponytail. He is tall and possessed of the awkwardness that sometimes goes with height, making him seem out of place in this ostentatiously cool penthouse. Tugging again at his collar, he fixes his attention on my neck. I'm wearing the flimsy blouse, its buttons done up all the way to the top, and a modest vest beneath.

"You're looking very—buttoned up," he tells me. It is the first time that anyone has really commented on my changed attire, and despite my careful buttoning and layering, I feel suddenly exposed. But he wasn't meaning to be unkind, and in the tricky silence that follows, he snaps into host mode, topping up my glass and flagging down more passing canapés. When an immaculate blonde in creamy cashmere and spike-heeled boots strides up to us, I assume we've been rescued. N sweeps his hand through his hair again, suggesting otherwise. The newcomer eyes me as she skewers a cocktail sausage.

"Are you his girlfriend?" she asks, nodding toward N. "Not that you'd know, of course. The last one didn't."

Afterward, installing the Beau in the spare room, I notice that the lint on his shoulder is in fact a small tear in his usually impeccable wardrobe. Closing the door and crossing the landing to my own room, I feel a pang of affection for this man with whom I've played romantic tag across several years and time zones. But I'm also relieved that he's sleeping where he is. Before, I'd have been too caught up in monitoring the currents of attraction between us to savor the tenderness in our friendship—the romance, really. It's possible that I took everything about him so personally, I never truly saw him until this evening. With my vow ruling out anything sexual, I'm able to appreciate our relationship as it miraculously still is, despite some tempestuous ups and downs. Eventually I will tell him all about my chaste endeavor, and he'll understand instantly a lot of what I find myself explaining to others. But that will come later; for now, I'm ashamed to say that I relish the secrecy of it, and the immunity—the advantage—it grants me in our usual game, where one of us seems always to be pursuing the other, heedless of the fact that we've never yet managed to coincide in our ardor.

The next couple of days breeze by, culminating in the dinner party that brings Mr. Vermilion and his bouquet to my door. Early the following morning, the Beau hauls his luggage downstairs, kisses me quickly on the cheek and is gone. From the airport, he sends a text, and without feeling compelled to sound it out for sexual resonance, I can take it for what it is: a thank-you for putting him up, chivalrous, fond and brushed with the bittersweet regret he is so good at. Standing barefoot in the kitchen, I experience all over again the elevation that those heels gave me. I'm so used to seeing sex as the story's climax, it hadn't occurred to me that our relationship might already be complete.

SEVEN

January OR *Sexual Sobriety*

Avoid stopping in for a drink after the theatre,
as the hour is a bit late, and it gives the young
man ideas. Don't fall for the old line of having
to go home for a long-distance call, and at the
very mention of works of art run in the
opposite direction.

—Alice-Leone Moats, *No Nice Girl Swears*

When it comes to romance, not even the most rational of us can resist conjuring omens and auguries from thin air. We read text messages like runes and stare into the bottom of our wineglasses as if they contain the wisdom of tea leaves. Perhaps it's simply that faced with so much irrationality (our own behavior can be baffling enough, never mind other people's), it seems only reasonable to tackle like with like. I know of one thirtysomething ad executive who by day manages giant budgets with skill and charm and by night tiptoes out into the moonlight to perform costly spells purchased from a white witch who has her own Web site.

I haven't tried magic, but I wish upon eyelashes, knock on wood and scan anxiously for second magpies (do they count as a couple if they're separated by streets or quarter-hours?). For this reason, I try to avoid astrology. Its followers revere it as a science, but it's my well-developed superstitious streak that it appeals to, and I worry that with just a little encouragement, my life would become cluttered with crystals and dream catchers before you could say "Age of Aquarius." Yet I can't help wondering whether people born into similar cultures at the same time of year mightn't share certain temperamental traits. That seems logical, doesn't it?

My own birthday falls early in January. Payback season for December's excesses, it's a cold month—generally the coldest in the calendar across the Northern Hemisphere (and in the Southern, the warmest)—though the days are getting lighter, and that light shines unforgiving on us when we topple from the resolution wagon. I've enough of a resolution to be getting on with already, but as another calendar page flips over, it occurs to me that my early-January birthday might have strengthened my belief in new leaves and fresh beginnings—in sparkling clean slates and wipe-down virtue. And if you believe in all that, then why wouldn't you license the occasional bout of bad behavior? My yoga-loving friend Krish, a lean vegetarian teetotaler whose calmness sometimes seems more chemical than Zen, once told me that birthdays are our own personal New Year. Because mine is so close to the real New Year, I get a double dose of giddily high hopes. It might also have given me a taste for extremes—made me into the kind of all-or-nothing type who renounces sex for a year, say. It's not quite that my birthdays and Christmases have always come at once, but I certainly grew up learning that good things come in a glut.

I saw in this New Year quietly, with my sister, my mum and rounds of manhattans—an apt-seeming cocktail for what is after all just the quarter-way mark in a very different year for me. In each there bobbed a maraschino cherry—a comic emblem of maidenly virtue, pickled in booze. And for my birthday? I don't throw a party, but I do gather friends in a bar. Getting ready in a rush in the loos at work, I pull a pair of tights from their packet only to discover that they aren't tights at all, they're stockings—not sticky-topped hold-ups, either, but the old-fashioned kind that require garters, a belt and a voluptuous manner. Dashing into a department store, I grab the nearest replacement pair and head to the bar.

A second set of loos, a second lot of hosiery—tights, yes, but in my haste, I've bought a toeless pair. Throughout the evening, I'm aware of the mini gusset separating my two big toes from their companions, digging in and reminding me of the elaborate ruses of concealing and revealing that we indulge in. Who would have thought there was even a market for toeless tights in the chill midwinter? My reactions make me feel frumpy, but I'm taking solace in the fact that for the first time since I embarked upon this journey, I have some abstemious company. Everyone seems to have given up something. January is a surprisingly good time for rallying friends, but just because they've shown up to raise a glass doesn't mean they plan on filling that glass with anything besides fizzy water. Most aren't drinking, a couple are on arcane detox diets and one seems to have given up speaking.

I alone have given up sex—unsurprising, you might think, except that humanity has a rich history of going without for set periods and ceremonial or sacramental purposes, as well as for more secular reasons. In ancient rites, periods of chastity were preludes to a renewal of energy—a new season, both figurative and literal. In Greece, for instance, the wives of Athenian citizens celebrated Thesmorphia, a three-day fertility festival, with abstinence. Held in honor of the goddesses Demeter and Persephone, it took the women off into the hills beyond the city, away from the prying eyes of their menfolk. There they reenacted the grief of Demeter, who created barren winter by renouncing her role as goddess of growth during the months her daughter was imprisoned in the underworld. For Demeter's Grecian worshippers, temporary renunciation of sex marked a pause for thanksgiving and paved the way for renewed fertility.

Postpartum celibacy is practiced by cultures around the world, from the North American Cheyenne to the Dani of Indonesia, functioning as a kind of birth control and improving the existing child's chances of survival. In Kaffa, the Ethiopian province that gave its name to coffee, it is believed that phases of celibacy in men increase their chance of fathering sons. The Catholic Church incorporates periodic celibacy into the rhythm method. In Judaism, sex is prohibited for some twelve days during and immediately after a woman's menstruation. Squeamish misogyny, you may think, but the traditional marriage contract explicitly states that at other times of the month, it is a man's husbandly duty to pleasure his wife.

Whatever else they may do, such proscriptions acknowledge a cyclical aspect of sexuality that is more in step with female desire. It's a notion that barely registers amid the sexual blare of current popular culture, in which the female form is depicted as constantly pert, receptive—up for it in a way that would cause outrage if their bodies were male.

While we still ritualize some temporary or cyclical sacrifices, sexless spells—drier than a teetotal January—are not among them, perhaps because we always feel they are forced upon us. If we did think it was as necessary as giving up caffeine or cutting out carbs, we'd be contradicting the contemporary view that sex is something it's impossible to get enough of—a tittering, teenage insistence on quantity over quality that glosses even chastity with sexual excess.

As several people have smirkingly told me these past few months, "Everyone will assume you had a *lot* of sex beforehand."

Self-control swung out of fashion with the sexual revolution. Just as virginity is now the preserve of mocked evangelical boy bands when once it was a vaunted vocation, crucial for protecting the rest of the community from avenging deities (consider the vestal virgins or their Incan equivalent, the Acllas), so we've come to regard celibacy as something almost shameful. This doesn't mean it's gone away, but it has gone underground—especially in the fraught context of a marriage. If there's a love that dare not speak its name in the twenty-first century, it is sexless marital love. As Aldous Huxley huffed: "Chastity—the most unnatural of all the sexual perversions."

One friend who didn't make it to my abstemious birthday celebration is Nina. My closest in terms of geography, she leads a life that is far removed in every other respect. In her late thirties, married and with a toddler in tow, she once worked fourteen-hour days producing telly shows about celebrity misadventures, and now she puts in the same hours ferrying two-year-old Alfie between play dates, naps and baby swimming classes. Except for when she escapes to meet me in the local café, which happens frequently because Nina luckily lives right around the corner. Unluckily, the café often seems to double as an unofficial crèche and is popular with dog walkers. The dogs and children share but a handful of names, and when someone yells "Digby" or calls out "Arthur" in a high-pitched, middle-class warble, you're never certain whether a golden retriever or a tow-headed child will come running. Both the mothers and the dog owners tend to scowl at Nina when she orders a glass of wine at four o'clock in the afternoon, no matter that Alfie is contentedly playing with packets of artificial sweetener while Digby/Arthur is running amok. What keeps us coming back, aside from proximity, is their chocolate torte—dark, and densely chocolaty in flavor, not just hue.

I'm eating the torte, enjoying the decadent kick as much as the cake itself, when Nina tells me that she'd like to set me up on a blind date with an old school friend of her husband's. I still remember the first time a setup was suggested to me. "He's a doctor," Priya had explained. I wasn't convinced. I wanted to know more—I wanted to know if he had nice eyes, a nice soul. Did he have hair? "He's not exactly *tall*," she admitted, before delivering the clincher: "If I were single, I'd be happy to be set up with him."

Matchmaking is a fraught business, bound to offend one party or the other. "So *this* is how she rates my smarts and charms," you think of your dear friend as the tubby guy in the elbowed pullover makes his way over to your table, looking as if he were thinking something very similar about you. But you can't refuse, not really. Long after those first few blind dates had slain any curiosity you may have had, you know that by turning the offers down—by refusing to even hear out the words "It's just a coffee!"—you're forfeiting your right to an audience when the next romantic banana skin sends you careening toward calamity. So when your friend asks, "What have you got to lose?" you pretend that the question is rhetorical, biting your tongue rather than rattling off the list that seems to grow longer with each successive date, beginning with self-respect, ending with self-respect, and in between cramming in everything from money to sleep.

Is the setup better than the online date? Well, you have someone to blame when it all goes wrong, but in all the worst ways, there is little to choose between them. Your mutual friend will have painted the verbal equivalent of the Match.com profile and mug shot, capturing the candidate's good angles, maybe winding back time a couple of years for good measure. Worse still, she'll have done the same for you. While he's some kind of brainiac stud—and just the sweetest, wouldn't you know it?—you'll have morphed into an Amazonian with Cordon Bleu skills and a bedroom smile. Oh, you'll be smart, too, if he asks, but somehow other traits will get mentioned first.

It also deprives you of the serendipitous element that is key to a really good how-we-met tale. Sure, you can still glance across the room, lock gazes, and *know,* but somehow shuttling e-mails back and forth, trying to hit on a time and a place that fits round his friend's stag night and your work crisis, isn't quite the same as both just happening to be right there, in the same moment. How many people still meet like that? One couple I know traded lingering looks, smoldering looks and finally words (a folded slip of paper was passed, like in a play or perhaps a classroom) in one of the world's most romantic places, the New York Public Library's Forty-second Street branch, but theirs is an increasingly rare story. For more and more couples, it starts with a click—a mouse click.

It is against all my better judgment, then, that I find myself listening to Nina as she describes the man she has in mind for me. I also tell myself this: I've already done lots of not having sex, but I've been neglecting the second part of my quest: the pursuit of love. Maybe, just maybe, this man will turn out to be my romantic destiny. "He's in a band," Nina is saying. "And he writes theme tunes and things—jingles, you know." Nina, I should point out, doesn't yet know about my year of chastity—I don't think she'd be trying to set me up if she did. I've been on the verge of telling her several times. I've always confided my life's messy romantic details to her, but *not* having sex seems an infinitely more private affair.

While trying to sell me on the jingle writer, she plays down his main advantage as a blind date: he's just moved into our postal zone. To get from my place to his, you'd walk down a big hill, dart across a confusing junction and look for a gap in the discount stores that line the main street. An alleyway leads to an improbably pretty mews, hemmed in by medium-rise blocks. It's not so close that we'll forever be running into each other, yet not so far that a bad date would squander an entire evening.

Over the phone, we settle on a pub that's midway between us. It's a cold evening when I head out, dressed in jeans and sneakers. It's partly my slouchy getup that makes the experience feel so new. Previous dates have been in places that suggest heels and lipstick. A city's topography can become haunted by past loves, but strangely, this patch of town—my own backyard—is virgin date territory. The men I've gotten involved with have tended to live in other neighborhoods, and we've always spent more time in theirs than in mine.

Pushing into the warm fug, I try to spot my date from the door. He texted me a few minutes ago to say that I'm looking for a man dressed in charcoal with a toad-green scarf, and I spot him almost immediately. He's tallish, with wavy hair and strong cheekbones. In one hand he holds a pint and in the other the scarf, which picks out the flecks in his hazel eyes. As I step toward him and he spots me, the unguarded youthfulness slips from his face, replaced by a smile that looks as relieved as my own feels.

Astonishingly, we get along. Two hours—three hours—slip by. We talk about reading and writing and trade neighborhood tips. We each mention exes in the way that you do—just in passing, to prove that even though you're single you're not a sociopath, and to prove that you're not hung up on them, that you're all set to move on. It's fun to be inside, drinking red wine and chatting on a damp, chilly night, but I can't forget that this is a date—that it's going well *for a date.* Of course, what happens at the end of a good date is a kiss, and after we leave the pub, he delivers me safely to the end of my road, where we stand awkwardly, both of us shuffling our feet, my eyes flitting nervously so as not to hold his pretty gaze for too long. Though kisses are allowed according to the rules of my year, the vow has made a kiss into a far greater event than it's been for a while. A kiss is now the first step on a path—a slippery one, I'm sure—that leads to the forbidden, and I'm reluctant to set foot on it lightly.

Do I really want to kiss him? In the context of this very pleasant evening, I can see that it's the thing to do, but here's the real thing: I don't think that I do want to kiss him. There is nothing wrong with him, and of course that in itself is exactly what's wrong. I should be able to list all that's astonishing, endearing, inspiring about him— all that makes me go weak at the knees—and yet I cannot. He appears to be thinking exactly the same, because he doesn't try for anything more than a peck on each cheek. Pushing his hands into his pockets, he flashes me a last smile and then turns on his heel.

Perhaps we just need to get to know each other a little. At least, that's the way I explain it to Nina. I've told her how well we got along, how much we found to talk about. I've admitted that, yes, he really is quite handsome. "But . . . ?" she asks, homing in on my unspoken doubts. "I don't know—I'm not sure there was a spark," I reply, though, to be honest, I'm not sure where I stand on "sparks" these days. After all, I had a veritable conflagration with Jake, and see where that got me.

Four days later, I meet him for a second date. Nudged forward in our diaries by busy weekends, its promptness feels keener than either of us feels, though in accordance with dating lore, we're escalating from drinks to dinner. A reservation has been made in a cheap-and-cheerful Thai local, and I'm making my way there straight from work, brandishing a mascara wand on a crowded bus, when he texts with a change of plan. The restaurant is deserted, he explains. "Want to go back to our regular?"

I have to walk past Plan A in order to reach Plan B and it is eerily empty, but expectantly so—like the setting for a surprise party, or perhaps just a really awful date. Back at the pub, I spot the Boy Next Door, this time sitting in the fancier dining section. He hasn't seen me yet and is looking out of the window, a trace of anxiety sharpening his features. My second first impression is more of the same—relief. His face has a delicate angularity—not feminine, but approaching beautiful nevertheless. Together we eat well, drink slowly and talk plenty.

It's a Tuesday night and the pub empties briskly, the shuffling others taking us with them. Like last time, he walks me home, and as we stroll up the hill, I can feel that awkward good-bye moment looming between us. My gaze grows furtive—I know what will happen if we maintain eye contact for too long. But if I don't kiss him now, will there be a third date? Will I mind? As if he has heard my thoughts, he begins telling me about a lecture on psychics that he's curious about, asking me if I'd like to go along. What should a third date be traditionally? A film? The quirkiness of his suggestion is so appealing that I nod yes.

The next afternoon, he texts to say there are no tickets left, but that he'll find us something else to do. I wonder if I'm leading him on. That I can't decide quite how I feel about him suggests yes. Then again, over the weekend I had a conversation with Becky about how surprised she is to find herself so happy right now with a man she met online. He's kind of nerdy, she told me, but after a couple of months she's grown attached to him. He makes her laugh and she feels like she can relax with him. She doesn't really like the sound of his voice, but that's okay, she added, neither does he.

It's not the Boy Next Door's voice that is my problem. Is it his teeth? Or maybe that strange overcoat he wears, that looks like it's been run up from an old tarpaulin but doubtless has a designer label stitched discreetly into one of its irregular seams? Truthfully, I can't pinpoint what's stopping me from falling for him, nor do I really want to; it's just that dating encourages us to pick away at each other—to become pickers even when we're not being picky. My instincts tell me that we're not a match, but I'm reluctant to trust them after so many outlandishly bad romantic calls. Would any of this be different were it not for my vow?

The following weekend, my sister tries to persuade me to join her in a crosstown trek to a klezmer-themed party in a nightclub. I feel momentarily rescued when a text pops up on my phone. It is the Boy Next Door, and he's in a pub—a different pub—right around the corner, watching soccer with some mates. Would I like to join them? he asks.

There are girls who like soccer and girls who pretend to like soccer, going along with their boyfriends. I frown at the message, wondering what could have given him the impression that I was either. At university, with Dan, I was one of the latter, but that was a long time ago. To anyone who knows me now, it would seem as outlandish a suggestion as the klezmer club—no, more so. Of course, he doesn't know me, but, then, what were we doing on dates one and two if not at least trying to get to know each other? Also, isn't it a little soon to be casting me in the role of soccer-watching girlfriend? It's nice that he wants me to meet his friends, but I'm not ready to sit beside him in silence with a pint and a bag of chips, waiting for halftime before he remembers I'm there. Candidly, what I'm craving is to be romanced a little more, and I think this does have something to do with my vow. Though the stakes are lower—I'm not going to sleep with him, right?—my expectations have grown higher.

Given that I've not been got by this man in the least, I realize I can get away with telling him that I'm heading west to an Eastern European rave. "Want to join?" I text back. A few minutes later, my phone chirrups: "I think out west might be a bridge too far." I agree—and I don't actually want to go, remember—but I'd wanted him to want to go. It's an unfair test, I know, but I need a sign that he's prepared to travel some distance for me—that we'd be edging toward a third date even if we weren't right on each other's doorstep.

Ten days later, Date Three finally rolls around. It's half past six on a Friday evening—a kind of witching hour: the streets are full of office workers shrugging off their weekday selves as they slip into bars or dive into underground stations. We're meeting at the British Museum to catch a late-night opening, and as I stroll through the gates and see its white pillars reaching up into the January night, I'm winded by the romantic potential of this place I've neglected the whole of my adult life.

In an e-mail, the Boy Next Door had first suggested we meet up in the Egyptian section, joking that he was a mummy's boy. The mummies were a focus of long-ago childhood trips, beloved by my little sister, squealed at by me. There was something about the smell of those rooms. Musky, too rich. And those poor urn-shaped mummified kitties—I'm not mad about cats, but the idea of any living creature winding up preserved for eternity as such a comically shaped package was just too sad. In the end, neither the Boy Next Door nor I could remember where the mummies were, so our rendezvous is set for the foyer, and here he is now, bending down in a rustle of strange gray coat and brushing my cheek with a kiss. Cold and slightly stubbly, it triggers a memory flash of other kisses from other men in other places.

The exhibition is crowded, and it's only once we've nudged our way near enough to the exhibit that I realize what we're looking at. Lining the walls are large photographs of desolate landscapes—sandswept, waterlogged, time-ravaged. On closer inspection, a pillar can be glimpsed here, some carefully laid-out foundations there. These are aerial views of lost civilizations. Surrounded by the encroaching wilderness, marooned by rising tides, they scream quietly of extinction. In a few of the photos, toy-size tourist buses can be seen, a detail somehow more depressing than all the ruined keeps and castles, cities and dreams, conjured up by the mounds of rubble.

Looking at art with someone you don't know well can be an uncomfortable experience. Our responses are so personal, there's no hiding the sudden gulfs in perception that open up as you stand before an abstract nude, for instance. The Boy Next Door is coping by making gags. I spot a fellow couple whose way of managing is simply silence. Yet another couple is smooching. Great, I think—nothing like a pair of smoochers to make the rest of us feel even more awkward. I turn back to the art just in time to come face-to-face with a photograph of chalk-and-pebble people scored into the surface of the earth, complete with pendulous breasts and penises that are surprisingly perky after all this time.

Next, we wander off to check out the mummies, all unchanged since I last saw them as a child. Maybe it's the excess of doom, maybe the cold that I can feel buzzing in my head, but I'd really like to be far away from here. It takes a bit of walking and a lot of optimism, but eventually we find a pub amid all the tourist "taverns." My wish granted, I consider the man sitting across from me. Those first two dates, I'd seen him before he saw me. This time round, he spotted me first. Composed, all primed for greeting, his face lacks the haunting delicacy that creeps in when he's caught unawares, and yet his eyes are such an appealing shade, his lashes so dark.

Where is this going? A quick drink to bring us back to life after all those lost civilizations, and then home alone? Already it has the feel of a long evening. Three whiskies later, I've used up all my anecdotes, yet I'm strangely happy to go on sitting here, gazing at his face.

"So where to next, whiskey girl?" It's a line that sounds borrowed from a film, or maybe he's quoting one of his own songs. His next line is probably being said across the city at this exact moment. "I have a bottle of wine back at my place."

As we drift in search of a cab together, I tell myself that it makes sense—he lives five minutes down the road from me, so it's almost as if I'm heading home. Still, I've a sinking feeling, and it's fitting that the pavements are now wet, the air rain-sodden. All around us, Friday nights are unraveling.

Heading south, we don't seem to have much to say to each other. "What are you doing?" a voice in my head screeches. The cab pulls up at his place and I end up paying most of the fare, so it's annoying that when he hands over my bills and his coins, he leaves no tip. Perhaps anticipation is making him careless. Of course he paid for the museum tickets and lots of that whiskey, but why am I even keeping tabs? Is he? Does there come a point when I owe it to him to explain my vow? Perhaps I should have told him right at the start.

This is a street I know well. I've even looked at a flat here myself and know before we step inside what the layout will be like. The

Boy Next Door moved in just a few months ago, and he takes my coat and hangs it on his newly nailed-up coat rack, gesturing toward a chair and explaining that his sofa is on order but won't arrive for another month. As he vanishes in search of the wine neither of us really wants, this thought crosses my whiskey-muddled mind: that I need to lower my property-purchasing standards and ramp up my relationship requirements. It's an unkind thought, and to make up for it I smile extra warmly when he wanders back in with two mugs of tepid white wine.

Though we're keeping at bay the silence that engulfed us in the cab, each new topic only widens the gulf between us. As if sensing this, he holds a hand out to me, reaching out across all that space, drawing me in to a kiss. My first kiss in five months. A kiss that sets me on a very dangerous downward slope. Actually, it's more dangerous than I'd thought, since it sends my mind reeling directly back to my last kiss, seasons ago now, back when the whole city was longing for rain and I was melting into Jake. That memory in turn yields to another, even longer ago—the magic of Jake's first kiss. All of this passes before me in a fraction of a second before the Boy Next Door's tongue returns me to the present kiss in hand. Having got embroiled in this, I should be giving more to it. A misplaced conscientiousness kicks in, and I catch myself wanting him to know that I can be good at this stuff—I want to do well and be liked, but while my tongue is in his mouth, my heart is far, far away. I may be hiding it from him, but I can't conceal it from myself. And then he says something that makes the comparison even more glaring. "You have a very kissable neck," he tells me, and I want to tell him that, no, my neck has already been claimed.

I don't, though I do somehow end the kiss and bring us back round to talking. I'd always thought such a rewind was impossible, but apparently not. Of course, this is the moment I should go home, but my thinking is crooked, and instead I'm listening to him describe a song he's written, all about famous corpses. This is just one dash of death too many for a single evening, and suddenly we're kissing again, tapping into a kind of pagan life force with renewed urgency. I try to think of all the good things about him, about how, looking at him earlier, I'd wanted to run my fingertips along these cheekbones, these eyebrows, about how cuppable his cheek had seemed. This time, I manage to lose myself—almost enough not to notice when my feet leave the floor as he holds me aloft for a second. Almost enough not to hear the small voice of my bigger self mutter that it's a very good job the sofa has been delayed, because after five months of abstinence, sofas possess seductively horizontal associations.

I'm not sure how long it lasts, but it's a pretty good kiss. When we come up for air, the Boy Next Door smiles coyly at me from beneath those long lashes and makes an announcement that promptly shatters any nascent spell.

"So, I'm being a best man in a few months, and the bad news is that I have to get up at nine o'clock tomorrow to help my friend shop for his groom's suit."

Given the treacherous blend of whiskey and whatever happy poppers are released during kissing, I'm surprisingly quick to realize what he's saying. He assumes I'll be staying over. It's dating by numbers and we're at number three. I smile inwardly.

Perhaps I should share something by Stendhal that I stumbled upon the other day. "A wise woman never yields by appointment. It should always be an unforeseen happiness," he writes in *On Love*. But that might sound too flirtatious, and I've misled us both enough.

"The really bad news is that I'm going home tonight, so you'll need to walk me up that hill fairly soon," I say instead.

I don't explain that as well as my mixed feelings for him, I've a nasty zit (he seems not to have noticed), a fluey feeling and some very unsexy knee-highs that will leave telltale rings around my calves, even if I were to manage to slip them off discreetly along with my heels. I definitely do not explain the vow that precludes all of the above.

Though it's only five minutes up the road, he elects not to walk me home, which isn't entirely surprising. Instead, he calls me a cab, pausing to kiss me in the hallway and do something that strikes me as far more presumptuous than his assumption that I'd be staying over: he smacks my bottom. I feel like I've stumbled into a British slapstick film of the *Carry On* kind. A moment longer, and out would pop Sid James. The cab up the hill costs £5 including tip, and as I let myself in through my front door, I remember a story I once heard about a friend of a friend who ranked men according to what the cab fare would have been had she returned to her bed rather than sharing theirs. If the alternative was a £35 ride home, clearly the guy was nothing special. If he lived just £10 away from her and still she chose to stay, he was probably a keeper—or at least someone she'd like to see again. It's one of those anecdotes whose neatness covers for its bleakness.

But what *was* I doing back there? What was I thinking, what was I feeling? I fall asleep happy to be alone but more aware than ever before of the full force of that word, and with the added problem of having led someone on weighing on my conscience.

The next morning, a shifty, slightly stubble-grazed face looks back at me from my bathroom mirror. A succession of quick-fire flashbacks return me to the night before, and that same question echoes: what was I thinking? Because I *was* thinking, even though I was trying not to, trying to go instead with the narrative flow and see where the evening led. Of course, I knew exactly where the evening was leading, and I knew that I wouldn't be able to follow its trail, not without breaking my vow. And what of my vow? Why didn't I simply tell him when I broke off that first kiss? In the wintry, early-morning light, blinking back at myself through splotches of toothpaste, I can see that sometimes, to not have sex is a far more personal matter than to have it. When faced with the challenge of explaining my decision to this man—this man who was so convinced that I *would* sleep with him—I realize that I don't know him nearly well enough, that the connections between us aren't nearly strong enough to risk offering him a glimpse of my inner self. Were I not vow-bound, I might have shown him plenty else instead. It would have had something to do with desire, but also politeness, amenability, an urge to please—a whole host of crazily misplaced sentiments. Or perhaps I wouldn't have. Perhaps I wouldn't even have gone on a second date, let alone a third, had it not been for the vow. Just as a nun's vestments grant anonymity, so my pledged chastity has begun to feel like a kind of invisibility cloak. It seemed protection enough to chance getting to know the Boy Next Door a little better. What I didn't realize is that it's actually my chastity that is invisible. Up until my hasty departure, nothing in my behavior had helped him to see it.

A few days later, I'm talking it over at Priya's birthday dinner. "He's not the one, then?" Neil says, sighing, next asking the really tough question, one he's never asked before: "So, if it's not him, who is this man you're looking for?" Seeing that his answer might be awhile coming, he puts it another way: "Okay, what kind of a book would he be?" A volume of verse, I decide. Superficially straightforward yet meaty enough to bear rereading. And Neil? He's looking for a thriller, he says, grinning at his partner, Ben, across the table.

They're a good couple, but there's a second reason for my smile. Though Neil's metaphor may not be much use out there in the dating world, it chimes perfectly with my great-aunt's romantic advice. She's always talked of men as books. "Take him back to the library," she'll say, if ever she disapproves of someone I'm telling her about. Appealing though it is, this idea of being able not only to browse but to borrow also probably belongs to a bygone era. Today, if you renew a "book" for a third time, it's pretty well assumed that you intend to read it all the way to the end.

It's only when I find an e-mail from the Boy Next Door that I realize I'd counted on not hearing from him again. It's a very sweet e-mail, inviting me round to dinner. He'd like to cook for me. This would be Date Four, and it would be starting at his place, never mind ending there. The sofa won't have arrived yet, but I glimpsed a perfectly serviceable bed on my way out last time. The irony is that he is offering precisely the kind of attention I was craving when I embarked upon this vow. He is treating me like a potential girlfriend rather than something sketchier. Fortified by my vow, my indecision has made it seem as if I've been playing hard to get. Game playing is something I've always scorned, but now I can't help acknowledging its effectiveness. It poses a question, too: would this invitation have materialized if I'd already slept with him?

EIGHT

February OR Romance on the Dance Floor

The fact of the matter is, it's very difficult to
tell love from passion. My advice to anyone
who doesn't feel sure of the difference between
them is either to give them both up or quit
trying to split hairs.

—James Thurber and E. B. White,
Is Sex Necessary?

As any nursery-school child clutching a crayoned card for "deer
mumie" will tell you, Valentine's Day falls on February 14.
But for plenty of solo souls, it comes round a lot sooner. My friend
Lucy, for instance, has been in a whirl of social planning for a full
fortnight already, first trying to convene single friends for cocktails,
then suggesting an actual cocktail party, and finally upgrading to
cocktails followed by dinner. It's the annual question: is it better to
suffer alone and hope that it passes quickly, or in company and risk
making too big a deal of it? Misery loves company, of course, though
having peaked so soon on the organizational front, Lucy is now
headed for an evening on her own, curled up in front of something
fluffy and masochistic like *When Harry Met Sally*.

Usually, my plan is to avoid it altogether or, if I can't help noticing

flower-stall inflation and the heart-shaped balloons bobbing in restaurant windows, to look the other way. After all, isn't it we who
expect the least of it who wind up making the most of it? Without
the likes of Lucy and me, anxiously, grumpily or perhaps hopefully
counting down, it wouldn't be such a *thing*. As it is, the spectacle we
make of ourselves must quicken the affection—and loosen the purse
strings—of anyone who has a someone.

This year is different; this year I'm making a token effort and
accompanying my sister to a singles party. A friend of a friend is
organizing it, and the date, February 10, reeks of pre-Valentine's
desperation. Its dress code is red or black—red for the romantics,
black for the cynics. I'm wearing a little black frock (with thick
tights, mind), a little black cardigan and a filthy black mood. As a
token gesture to the bighearted optimists, I have scarlet nails. I'm
also wearing mean red heels in which I fully intend to trample any
misguided romantic who strays my way. One additional detail: on
my finger is the New York ring, to remind myself that I'm not a real
cynic, not yet, just a Valentine's Day cynic. Make red everything
that's black in my outfit, and you'll have a fair idea of what my up-
beat sister is wearing. Though we're quite different, our differences
have a habit of unifying us. We're opposite sides of the same coin.
You'd definitely spot that we were sisters, and right now, walking
down the street together, the two of us look as if we've raided Beryl
the Peril's wardrobe.

We take the bus there, and my mood lifts a little. I'd forgotten
how contagious it can be, the excitement of joining that hope-filled
Saturday procession, all on our way Out—out into the velvet-skied,
twinkly night, where who knows what enchantment might await.
Everyone is dressed up; the air is scented with perfume and after-
shave and hair spray. Gaggles of girls link arms as they totter along;

men's silhouettes are origami-crisp, their freshly ironed shirts worn untucked, their hair slick with product.

The club's name, Mint, smacks of a chain of lap-dancing clubs but apparently derives from *minted,* which its founders were before opening up and, doubtless, discovering how costly it can be to enable people to have a good time. Giving our names to the bouncer, we step toward a long, dimly lit corridor of a room. Booths line its length, and at the far end a bar gleams. A handful of men and one woman are clustered with drinks, their conversation so hushed it's inaudible above the whispery tunes that congeal in the darkness. They are the only other people here.

As we perch on bar stools, sipping cocktails called U-pimps and chatting to the girl—an irrepressibly perky headhunter, it turns out—the club slowly fills up. It's an unlikely crowd for a central London club on a weekend. Mostly finance folk, the men in their late thirties or early forties and the women a few years younger. Though clearly single—why else subject yourself to this?—they have the round-edged look of practiced players. The men are in the kind of jeans bought by people who spend their lives in suits; the women favor pretty chiffon floral print dresses probably intended as country wedding attire.

To begin with, it is exactly like a school dance—the original school dances, back when we were eleven, say, boys on one side of the room, girls on the other. Our new friend is all business. Having already found out what my sister and I do, she says we'll be hits when we reveal that we're so arty. "Bankers love arty women," she insists. For herself, she's used to men being nice purely so that she'll find them new jobs for free. As I reach the bottom of my drink, fishing out a vodka-plumped blackberry before my glass is whisked away, it occurs to me that if she's right, men would only be doing what powerless (but not guileless) women have resorted to for centuries—using sex as leverage. The idea of a Square Mile teeming with male Becky Sharps is quite appealing.

While television schedules and bookshop displays testify to our fascination with sex that's for sale, the more humdrum commerce of intercourse—a commerce presumably even older than the world's oldest profession—has become mildly shocking. Promising sex in return for mowing the lawn or minding the kids on a Saturday morning? Well, it's just not very enlightened, is it? And if selling sex to get what you want appears plucky and puts you in line for a blogged-about blog, then withholding it for the same end seems merely manipulative. We're tolerant of or else avidly interested in the boob jobs of aspirant C-listers—women with apparently zero interests or ambitions beyond their own implanted, stylized sexual allure—tracking them in the red tops and weekly gossip mags as they trade up from dating a reality TV star to a spoiled celeb scion to a Premier League soccer player. Yet the very idea that a woman might deploy wiliness and premeditation and parlay her virtue into anything as mundane as a wedding ring—why, it's an outrage!

In 1740, Samuel Richardson published one of the first modern English novels, a two-volume epistolary tome based on a true tale that he claimed to have heard from a "gentleman." *Pamela: or, Virtue Rewarded* describes the travails of its eponymous heroine, a fifteen-year-old servant whose bad luck it is to catch the eye of her employer's son, a squire named "Mr. B." Resisting his advances, she escapes the fate of many a real-life maid—pregnancy, dismissal, ruin if not death—by dint of her determination and resourcefulness. Despairing of finding a way to bed her, Mr. B eventually proposes, and she goes on to become the darling of the bluebloods.

"No man can understand why a woman shouldn't prefer a good

reputation to a good time," wrote Helen Rowland in her 1903 memoir, *Reflections of a Bachelor Girl*. She'd be dismayed to learn that the very idea of a good reputation has since become history. Or perhaps she wouldn't; perhaps she'd recognize it as a yoke we've done well to throw off. The problem is, we've replaced it with another. Today's "bachelor girl" is expected to want sex constantly, and is primed to invest money, time and other equally finite resources, like patience and hope, in its pursuit. But what of the people who just aren't that into it? And what of those who really do love sex—enough to keep it special?

The question of how to create value for something that no longer carries mainstream currency has preoccupied Christian youth movements in recent decades. Father-daughter "Purity Balls" (sometimes more queasily known as "Purity Weddings") ritualize the moment at which a girl pledges to remain a virgin until marriage, protected by her father, while teen members of groups like True Love Waits wear rings to symbolize similar vows. The criticisms are considerable, and range from concerns about young girls losing custody of their own latent sexuality to statistical evidence suggesting that not only do most break their vows, but when they do, they tend to take fewer precautions.

A common metaphor used by supporters depicts virginity as a gift that cannot be rewrapped. Once opened, however hard you try to wrap it up again, you'll always be presenting a gift in crinkled paper. The main flaw in this parable is its distracting emphasis on the paper. If a recipient cares that much about the gift wrap, he probably doesn't appreciate you. But fixating on virginity doesn't really help, either. Virginity is, after all, a default state. Once you've presented it to your husband, tied with red ribbon, or else squandered it on the class lothario behind the bike shed, you're off the hook. To live chastely is a more enduring commitment.

Richardson's *Pamela* went through five editions in its first year. It also inspired numerous parodies, most notably Henry Fielding's *Shamela* and its sequel, *Joseph Andrews,* in which gender roles are reversed and Shamela's brother, a footman, finds himself harassed by his rapacious employer, Lady Booby. For all their picaresque satire, Fielding has a point to make: Richardson's heroine was a sham, he says. She cared less about her virtue than about the price she could exact for her virginity. Real virtue was not for sale. Today, its market has vanished. As Mae West quipped, "Don't keep a man guessing too long—he's sure to find the answer somewhere else."

While we oversell sex, we don't seem to value it. It is too readily available, just another disposable commodity—a simple case of supply and demand, as any of the bankers now circling our headhunter friend would explain. Devalue the word *no* and the market is flooded, causing *yes* to depreciate simultaneously. Perhaps part of the fascination of the hooker—and the courtesans and geishas who preceded her on the best-seller lists—is that she dares to put a price on sex. After all, we can get in touch with our inner whore just by flipping through the pages of a glossy magazine. The hooker, even as she cheapens her wares, does at least give them some kind of value.

As the bartenders step up their pace and empty glasses are traded for second drinks and thirds, the room's gender divide begins to blur. The male half seems emboldened by something else besides U-pimps: being here at this particular party signals our desperation as surely as *single* means "available." It makes us fair game and it makes our suitors keen. Why would a man want to date a desperate girl? He wouldn't; we're just witnessing the unspoken side of being officially single: romance may be our object, but sex seems to be the currency.

Lots of people already know one another from work, it transpires.

If they've been seeing one another daily and still haven't grabbed that drink or quick bite together, how keen can they be? "Maybe they just need an icebreaker," my sister suggests, shaking her glass. "You know, a change of scene." We take in the decor, which is retro bachelor pad, circa *American Gigolo*. It doesn't bode well for the longevity of any resulting relationship.

Meanwhile, a whole layer of social veneer has been stripped off, pages of preamble torn out. One guy walks up to me. "What kind of a man are you looking for?" he asks. There's no "Who are you?" It's all "Whom do you want?"

"Oh, you know—the usual," I tell him. "Smart, funny, handsome." I laugh, because it sounds like an awful lot this evening. Even two out of the three feels a tall order, and it's lucky I'm not fussy about height.

I haven't been to one of these events in such a long time, I can't tell if it's just my vow making me extra sensitized. Why am I putting myself through this? At least for some of these others, sex is a viable reward, a fleeting consolation for putting yourself out there. My friend Neil told me recently about how he watches colleagues at the charity where he works head off on dates with people they've met online. He's the kind of man you want to confide in—a good and wise listener with a warm brown gaze, though my theory is that his confidability has more to do with his ears, which stick out like a cartoon schoolboy's and must have flagged down every playground bully. Whatever you are about to tell him, those ears say, he has probably been on the receiving end of worse. Either way, his colleagues creep into work the next morning, and before lunchtime will have unburdened themselves to him. For all the colorful variation of their stories, he says that essentially they boil down to this: either they slept with their date—their first date—and feel lousy about themselves, or they didn't sleep with their date and feel rejected.

After less than an hour at the party, I am desperate for just one thing: to leave. I'm pretty certain that my sister is having as cheerless a time but she is a glass-half-full girl, even when that glass contains a porny-sounding cocktail of despair and opportunism.

"Twenty minutes longer," she says.

"Ten," I counter, figuring it'll take us that long to work our way through what has by now become a heaving crowd.

It's as we're shuffling toward the door that we become wedged beside three guys, dressed head-to-toe in black and making less effort than even we are to talk to anyone but one another. Later, one of their group—Raj, who is in real estate though dreams of breaking into the Indian music scene, or so he says—will explain that it was our sulkiness that appealed. I suppose, exit-bound, we look safely not on the pull. Raj's friends are Rafiq, who is about to launch an online art gallery, and Jean-Christophe, who is Belgian and very jet-lagged, having just flown in from a place whose name I don't catch. Before we know it, a bottle of pink champagne has materialized.

We stay, of course, and our band of five edges toward the dance floor. The whispery refrain of our arrival has been usurped by a throbbing beat that occasionally gives way to teasing snatches of vocal melody.

"You know I want to fuck you," croons an androgynous voice as the lights dip lower, plunging the club into near darkness. All around us, incongruously dressed singles are busting MTV moves, and mimicking badass raunch. Their performances seem mimed, and rather than intimating hidden sexy depths, the effect is panto-mimic, almost neutering.

Not that this is safe territory for wallflowers, either. As soon as she sits down, my sister is approached by a paunchy man in a scarlet shirt. Robin Redbreast gives up on conversation almost immediately—due partly to her lack of interest (total but polite), but mostly, it seems, to the fact that he's positioned himself directly beneath a speaker. Only when he gets up do we spot that he's also wearing earplugs. He clearly didn't come here to chat.

"They're all looking for love," Rafiq observes. If he was aiming for irony, it is drowned out, but instead I hear a kind of melancholy truth. Most would probably agree that that is indeed what they want, and few would doubt their own sincerity. But who would search for love in a place where it's too loud to hear and too dark to see? I suppose the powerful musk of sex—so easily confused with love and so simple by comparison—throws us off the scent. After all, this party was billed as a warm-up for that great romance fest, Valentine's Day, yet sex is what is on offer. It's there in the music and on the drinks menu, and, just to make us women feel really frumpy, it's embodied by the lithe young cocktail waitresses—none is over twenty, all are skinny and blond. Dressed in leggings and skirts so abbreviated they'd look more clothed without them, they slink between the gyrating fund managers on regulation three-inch heels, drink-laden trays held aloft.

Once upon a time not so very long ago, dating took place in the female sphere. Men would come a-calling, and a strict etiquette governed their visits. Then courting couples started stepping out, and if they stopped for an ice cream cone, the men picked up the tab. When the motor car arrived, it offered a private space—with a backseat on which a young woman might demonstrate her gratefulness. While that backseat quickie might have led to marriage (or, let's not forget, a terrifying backstreet abortion), a girl is nowadays lucky if a night spent "rummaging," as one male friend of mine so delightfully puts it, wins her a telephone number or a cup of tea the next morning. Gone is courtship; here to stay, it seems, is "the mating game" and all its testosterone-drenched terminology.

Still, to prove that restraint hasn't made a prude of me, and to show some solidarity with these lonely-hearted seekers, I get up and join the dancers. In a corner, a group of cool girls are demonstrating that they actually can dance, though their skill and unity seem to be repelling men—that and their withering looks. "Met anyone?" yells one of them. I nod vaguely toward the pink champagne table. "Anyone you'd seriously consider?" she adds, laughing raucously when I throw the question back at her. "Well, you've got to get out here, otherwise you don't know what you're missing, right?" Clearly reassured that she's missing nothing, she leads her posse prancing off in the direction of a fish tank, whose inhabitants they proceed to scrutinize with far more interest than they've shown any of the bankers.

Rafiq has shimmied over by this point. He fits his body close to mine, limboing us earthward and then up again as we cling to a few bars of something semirecognizable. Is he feeling what I'm feeling? That we're going through motions so well rehearsed we've forgotten their meaning? Then again, my vow acts as a constant reminder of that meaning, and it isn't exactly chaste. Railing against waltzing in his 1893 *Ladies' Guide in Health and Disease,* John Harvey Kellogg quoted "Prof. Welch," a popular dancing master from Philadelphia. "Dancers of to-day come in altogether too close contact," the instructor admonished. "In the olden time a gentleman merely touched a lady's waist, at the same time holding her right hand in his left. Now he throws his arm clear around her form, pulls her closely to him, as though fearful of losing her, brings his face into actual contact with her soft cheek, and, in a word, hugs her." Kellogg, who frankly considered Welch a little too forgiving in his assessment of

the waltz, also noted that New York's chief of police had cited dancing as the cause of ruination for three-quarters of the city's "abandoned girls."

Because I'm here—and because there's nothing like the idea of
transgression for adding fizz to tired moves—I loosen up enough to
start having fun. And this is fun! When was the last time I went dancing? I've a glass of pink champagne in my hand and—oh! Just then, a
crash breaks above the thrusting music and suddenly the dance floor
is sequined with shards of broken glass. Was it my hand that collided
with the passing tray? A waitress vanishes like a bunny in a puff of
tiny skirt. Almost immediately, the dancers close back over the spill-
age, but not before Rafiq has gently, precisely kicked the stray fragments safely beneath a banquette. It is the first sign I've seen all
evening that romance might still have a pulse in it. It's chivalrous, is
what it is, and who am I to scorn chivalry? If sex is the consolation
prize for everyone else here tonight, I'll claim chivalry as mine.

We leave shortly afterward, me, my sister and our pink-champagne-
bearing knights. On my way to the cloakroom, I catch the eye of the
headhunter, who flashes an I-told-you-so smile of approval.

We lose the Belgian, but as a foursome head off in search of one
last drink. It feels like we've survived something together, and we're
not ready to part quite yet. We trade stories about exes and weigh
up speed-dating and the Internet as alternatives to singles parties.
Rafiq tells us about a New York import that recently set up shop in
London—a matchmaking bureau to which men may sign up only if
they're earning in excess of x—an extra-large X—amount each year.
He isn't sure what the qualifications for women are, but we all agree
they probably involve a photograph rather than a bank statement.

It's long past midnight by the time we step out into a fine drizzle.
My heart sinks as two competing packs of bedraggled partygoers

dash by in pursuit of an empty cab. Luckily, Raj claims to have a chauffeur. I don't really believe him, but I'm suddenly so eager to be home asleep that I can't bring myself to entirely disbelieve him, either. Maybe I spend too much time with struggling artistic types— maybe every real estate tycoon has his own chauffeur. We shelter in the doorway while he mumbles into his mobile phone, and sure enough, a few moments later a car pulls up to the curb.

It seems more like a personal minicab than a chauffeur service— where are the driver's epaulettes and cap, my sister wants to know— but we're not quibbling, not at all. We're dry, warm and homeward-bound. And if a pumpkin can become a carriage—well, then, perhaps a tame minicab can be a chauffeur-driven car and a party full of loneliness become a ball in memory, a joyous evening on which we danced, drank pink champagne and were escorted home by two charming princes. Perhaps this is the trick with romance, too. Perhaps, like good sex and fairy tales, it is partly in the mind—in how you choose to spin it the next morning. Waking up alone gives you that scope—the scope to decide what kind of a story you'll tell. Meanwhile, the presence of Raj's "chauffeur" makes it very simple indeed not to invite them in for coffee.

I still have on my token red-for-romance nail polish come February 14, and it flashes at me as I go about my day. In the library, it leaves scarlet scuffs on the pages of books—faint, illegal. The hush in the reading room is usually charged with stolen glances and erotic daydreams, but not today—today, it seems like a refuge for the romantically scorned, who fill row upon row, heads determinedly down, their thoughts wrestling with those of the author baring all on the page in front of them. Will this be the sum of their day's intimacies?

I stay till the rush hour has ebbed, stepping out into a cold, rain-smeared evening. Crossing the courtyard, I pass a friend hurrying in, barely hidden excitement in his eyes. I hope he's headed toward an assignation in there. Stopping by the supermarket, I catch the last-minute crowds of men buying bouquets of mismatched left-overs, anxious looks on their faces. Back at home, there are no flowers, no cards. Not that I was expecting anything. After all, I dismissed my one suitor, the Boy Next Door, a few weeks ago, turn-ing down his dinner-for-two offer with a polite, cowardly few lines. "Busy at work, in a strange place right now, lovely invitation but . . ." We all know the script. What I do find is an e-mail from a friend forwarding a last-minute party invitation. Its dress code is "decay-ing beauty" and its decadent attractions include the world's weepi-est music, Fado. "I'll be there peeling onions at midnight," he writes, having outed us all as the loveless at the top of his message—no tactful blind copying today. For a moment, I'm half tempted. I feel a flicker of the emotion that electrified my twenties—the sense that I might be missing something.

Instead, I go to bed with a pile of books. When I wake, it is Feb-ruary 15. It is also two A.M., the lights are still blazing and my cheek is stuck to the page of a novel. This diet of fiction—it can't be healthy. But before I can reflect any more, I notice a message glim-mering on my BlackBerry. It's from the Beau. He's on New York time, he tells me, meaning that it's still the fourteenth and he can legitimately wish me a happy Valentine's. He adds a shared joke that we've kept going for years, all about where we'd run away to for a weekend together, suggesting that we ditch Iceland in favor of a hotter destination. Senegal, perhaps. It's meaningless, really, but it's one of those in-jokes that demonstrate what intimacy is all about. In past years, I've fixated on being alone, but real intimacy doesn't require physical proximity, just as physical proximity doesn't guarantee intimacy. More than anything, the Beau's message is a reminder of the day's utter artificiality and its real magic. Sometime, somewhere, it will always be February 14.

How do you dress for a business meeting with a man you met at a singles party? At some point during that red and black evening, I'd got to talking to Rafiq about work—his, mine, whether we might be able to do something together. It was in that context that I heard from him the following day, a perfectly worded e-mail that somehow managed to recall all that we'd said and very little of the backdrop.

It's not a straightforward decision, but as I haul myself up onto a seat at the bar, I realize that picking out the right pair of trousers to match the right smart yet insouciant top was the easy bit. It's knowing whom to be that is hard. Beside me a collection of props seems to offer a clue—an ideas-filled notebook, a press release bearing some circled facts—but when I open my mouth, something is missing from my voice: a note of confidence that I can usually count on hearing, if not feeling.

Rafiq had suggested dinner, and in commuting it to lunch, I'd thought I was clarifying things, but here we are in a windowless bar so dark it could be midnight. It's a hotel bar, and though we'll shortly be heading through to the restaurant, something in the staff's extreme tact suggests that we might as well have booked ourselves a room for the afternoon. They're simply taking our coats, jotting down our drinks order, requesting a reservation name, yet their hushed delicacy positively shrieks assignation.

My awkwardness doesn't improve much when we're seated back

in what passes for daylight, staring out through picture windows at joggers trudging around the grayish park.

"This isn't an interview," Rafiq begins when the waiter is finally done explaining the specials. "But it's not a date, either. I just thought it would be nice to spend some time getting to know you while we went through the work stuff—even if it's just as friends." He punctuates himself with a laugh that sounds like a cough, and I wonder if I'm in for something rehearsed. What follows is about as clear as the sky outside, from which a misty rain is now falling, yet somehow, the mere acknowledgment of a personal subtext sets me at ease. That note of confidence I was missing earlier on—was it sexual confidence?

Time drifts pleasantly and lunch draws to a close. At one point, we find ourselves exchanging broad grins without much reason, locking gazes for just a little too long. Just as well this isn't dinner, I think, as Rafiq lays his credit card on top of the discreetly folded bill. He drives me home in a low-slung, ridiculously flashy sports car, through one park and then another, where we get lost and find ourselves spiraling in slow, shrinking circles toward its green center. I'm already looking forward to saying good-bye so that I can play it all back in my mind.

But there's something I'm not telling you. On my way to lunch, I sent a text to Jake, the first contact I've had with him since that August day—his birthday—more than six months ago. My premise was an invitation from my sister to a film screening she's organizing. It's the next day. As the little envelope somersaulted off into the ether, I wondered whether I'd been rash—but not for long, because the rush of having done it was too great. What am I playing at? you might wonder. Well, until I hit SEND, I'd have said I was merely trying to prove to myself that I'm over him. I need to see us for what we were rather than what I was yearning for us to become, and I finally feel ready. That post-send rush, though—it's worrying, especially when he texts back saying that, yes, he'll be there.

I ask along Rafiq, too, though in the end he doesn't make it. He sends a faultlessly friendly text, apologizing that he has to spend time with his nephew—a sure point-winner. Still, even in absentia he is a helpful distraction. It's his possible arrival that I train any spare anxiety on, so when Jake finally walks through the door, I'm swept into a tight hug before I've really had a chance to register that it's him. It's with my face pressed into his neck that the knowledge makes its way to my brain, but by then it's too late—the rest of my body knows. The physical flashback is jolting. After all these months, the shock of skin-on-skin contact with him leaves me doubting my resolve as he turns and heads for the auditorium. Maybe Kellogg's dancing instructor had a point—a hug *can* be a girl's undoing.

Inside the small, plush cinema, most of the seats are already taken. The front row is empty except for Jake, alone at the far end. With my sister waiting for me to sit down so she can signal to the projectionist to get things rolling, there's nothing for it: I head for his row. The lights dim, and for the next forty minutes, while my sister's film surrounds us with experimental sound and staccato images, I'm conscious mainly of the person sitting a whole six empty seats away, one velvety square for each of the months I've tried to put between us.

After the applause and the Q&A, the milling audience brings us together. Jake is putting on his best boyish act—bright, persuasive. Clinging to the idea of this encounter as a chance to prove to myself that I'm over him, I chatter on, unwilling to confront any intensity that our silence may still carry, yet asking none of the questions that I tortured myself with when we were involved. Not asking, for instance, if he's finally broken up with his girlfriend. It's only when he says again, pausing for emphasis, how nice it was to find my text after all that time that I stop talking long enough to listen. Do I hear hurt in his voice?

The crowd has thinned and we're drifting toward the Saturday bustle beyond by the time he suggests dinner, a chance to catch up properly. "Or lunch?" he adds. And there it is again, that choice between two meals whose menus conceal such different messages. His smile is casual, but there is hope in his eyes and I force myself to look away.

"Lunch," I say quickly, before I'm able to change my mind. Instantly he begins prevaricating, telling me next weekend, then adding that he'll have to make some phone calls first—relatives visiting from out of town, work.

Should I have answered neither lunch nor dinner but coffee? Should I have left it at neither? Yet the invitation is a tacit acknowledgment of the unasked questions and unexplained answers that have been weighing on our pleasantries. Perhaps their asking and explaining—over lunch, just lunch—will grant me the closure that I'd hoped to attain today by simply seeing him.

His scent hovers round me for the rest of the afternoon—ornate, seductive, but more basic than either of those refined words suggest. It beckons me back to analyze his every word and gesture, to wonder if anything has changed. Yes, I remind myself, something has changed—I have changed. All the same, I can't help thinking my vow has at last met its real challenge.

NINE

March OR *Swooning to Conquer*

Every kiss, like a gulp of wine, added to the
warmth of her body. Every kiss increased the
heat of his lips. But he made no gesture to
raise her dress or to undress her.

—Anaïs Nin, "Hilda and Rango," from *Little Birds*

've been waiting for Jake to cancel. I even tried to make it easier. "Maybe some other time?" I texted, hazy, unspecified. Lunch day swings round and brings neither cancellation nor confirmation. Irritatingly aware of that old hold he has over me, I clump around the house, pulling on jeans, cowboy boots, a cardigan with almost military detailing—nothing soft. A headache hovers, which is why I reach for the perfume that I still think of as his: it's a lighter scent, I tell myself, less likely to trigger a migraine. It is almost noon when my phone bleeps—he's running late but he's made a reservation.

A reservation.

Suddenly my breezy lunch is looking a lot less casual. Could I be in trouble here? I peer outside, looking for some kind of divine sign, or at least a clue as to whether or not I'll need an umbrella, but things seem capricious, early blossoms swaying beneath cloud-scudded blue.

The restaurant is of the kind where you pay to sit a long way away from everyone, including your dining partner, and its crisp tablecloths lure in the day's brightness. Distracting myself with the menu, I don't notice Jake until he's standing in front of me, stooping to hug me and offering greetings, apologies, excuses. I take in neither his words nor his nearness, it's all too quick; and now here he is, sitting at an almost safe distance across from me. His charm is switched to full blaze and he's as sleek as ever, but the cleanness of his shave and the dampness of his hair make him look just a little defenseless, too. *Naked* is the word, and it's one I'm trying very hard to unthink.

What we talk about, I couldn't really tell you—he mentions his girlfriend at one point and I wince inwardly. I think of telling him about my chaste year, then think again and stop at the mention of a "project." The rest of our chat is bland, his inquiries polite, my responses solicitous. We're just trying to keep that silence at bay and stay away from the edge of the liquid chasm that pools between us when our eyes meet for too long—which truthfully is anything more than a heartbeat. And yet we're not hurrying. Gradually the restaurant empties around us. Our two courses have come and gone and the waiters have relaxed, their postures slackening; an off-duty laugh sounds from somewhere behind the scenes. Midway through mint tea, Jake slips out to top up the parking meter, buying us extra time in which we drift together, becalmed amid those blank midafternoon hours that seem to exist only at the weekend. Despite the dazzling white tablecloths, it's clear that outside the light is changing, a reminder that the day's spring notes were illusory after all. Meanwhile, our gazes are growing bolder, our words fainter, and still neither of us seems inclined to reach for a jacket or scrape back a chair—to make the first move. Instead, Jake makes a move of a kind that's altogether more familiar: he holds out his hands, palms up. An invitation, but to what? To take solace in our shared might-have-been? A sentimental squeeze for old times' sake?

It's then that I catch the soundtrack. It must have been there all along, inaudibly flavorless, buried in the background clatter of cutlery and Saturday cheer. The song that snakes around us is not flavorless. It begins with those bluesy, languid piano chords, the bass fooling around below while Erma Franklin, Aretha's big sister, sweetly asks whether she ever held anything back from her man. Next, the chorus sashays in with its sighing lament, oohing and aahing in sympathy, until a drumroll ramps it all up, and before you know it you're caught in the embrace of a big-souled ballad, with Erma belting it out, showing her no-good lover just how tough a woman can be. "Piece of My Heart" has an indomitable spirit, uptempo even in the face of such plainly told despondency. Yet for all its feisty encouragements to take control of your heartbreak, to own it, the backing singers give the song away for what it really is: an exquisitely masochistic come-on to abandon yourself to love's sweet hurt, to glory martyrlike in its achy-breaky rapture. It is irresistible.

You see where this is going, don't you? For a while—at least a verse of Erma—I try to pretend that I haven't noticed Jake's hands, proffered so invitingly. I feel my grip on my teacup tighten, and beneath the table, I'm channeling nervous energy into frantic foot-tapping. Noise seems to be doing something odd, too. My heart is racing, my cheeks feel flushed—no, my entire body feels flushed, oversensitized. Oh, I'd like to blame the soundtrack. That would be wrong, though it's true to say that without Erma's catchy exhortations to "Take it!" my own hand might have stayed safely on its proper side of the table. Instead, it stretches out and strays into the no-man's-land of the sugar bowl, the salt cellar.

It takes Jake's.

This is fine, I tell myself, we'll just sit here holding hands, bidding good-bye to whatever enchantment was, and now no longer is. It's companionable, noble even. It's the scene we should have had right at the start—our "there's too much in the way" moment. Wait, it's *Brief Encounter*!

The voice inside my head gabbles on like Dolly Messiter, that awful busybody in the film, but really, I know I am lost—I know as much even before I look into his eyes and our lips meet, before the kiss hits my system. And there's Erma—she can't stand the pain, but then she goes ahead and gives in and off they go again. The instant our fingertips touch, the world recedes in a rush. It's just the two of us, just the warm pressure that isn't pressure at all, more like its opposite—weightlessness. I'm floating, so as we lean into our kiss, it comes as a surprise that my body still needs to strain a little to bridge all that white linen. As it does, I feel the distance that I've striven to put between us these past months vanish—covered sooner than you could say "Take it"; swifter than you could beg "Break it."

When I was growing up, our repertoire of treats included packets of paper flowers from a Chinese shop, bright scrunches that unfurled when set sail in a saucerful of water. The afternoon is unfolding with a similarly vivid, slow-motion inexorability. We're standing outside, pressing into each other, oblivious of time, place, passersby. I'm sliding into Jake's car, edging through streets in a direction that I know so well—the opposite direction to home. His apartment seems smaller than I remember it, as if I've grown since I was last here, which in a way I have, though it's what remains the same that is so disorientating. Even ephemera like light and ambient noise seem to be direct echoes of so many other moments here with Jake.

It's when we're stretched out on his sofa together, face-to-face, that I feel almost weepily overwhelmed. My head doesn't stand a chance against this sensory overload. The sight of him—his face is a face I could look at forever; the feel of his lips tingling still on mine; the scent of him. It's the scent that really gets me. Time concertinas and I'm right back in the place his presence always takes me to, feeling both lost and found, hope-filled and hopeless. I'd been so certain that I was over him—but not so certain that I hadn't felt the need to prove it to myself. If only I'd resisted that urge to know for sure. Could it be that I'm about to get under him once again?

Except that no—this time there's the matter of my vow. But how do I go about halting something I've never cared to interrupt before?

Our kisses are so complete, so all-encompassing, that I'm not immediately aware of what Jake's hands are doing. They're roaming. Roaming with intent, going places no man's hands have gone in a long while. In almost eight months, in fact, and those hands—they were Jake's, too. With that thought, the sweet nostalgia of it all sours, because as surely as I know where this is going in the breathless here and now, I also have a keen idea of where it's headed in the long term—nowhere, certainly not if I let myself behave in the exact same way as last time.

It's an immense act of will, but I stay Jake's hands long enough for the heat to cool a few degrees.

"I can't do this," I tell him. He freezes—as much out of surprise as from any implied command—and for a split second, I'm as curious as he seems to be about what I'm going to say next. Stretched out on his sofa, we're lying so close together our voices sound loud even as we whisper, our words becoming oddly corporeal—all tongues and teeth, each one weighing so much in the dusky air.

"The project I mentioned earlier . . ." I've begun, and the only way is onward. "It's a vow of chastity. A year-long vow of chastity."

There, I've said it. My cheeks are hot—why is it that the *c*-word keeps making me blush? But now that it's out in the open, I'm feeling defiant—I've stopped the rerun of our story in its tracks. While almost every fiber of my body wishes I hadn't, it's given me an exhilarating taste of something entirely new: control. But now it's Jake's words that I'm hanging on. He is the first man I've told in these circumstances, and how does he react? He laughs.

No, he guffaws.

It's a cartoon bubble of a guffaw, all exclamation marks and unpronounceable vowels. I don't hear unkindness, more like a full appreciation of the absurdity of the situation: as if he hadn't already put enough obstacles in our way, I'm now adding an enormous one of my own. And while I blush saying "chastity," I've noticed that it makes others uncomfortable, too. There's something oddly titillating about the notion—as if we've all heard so much about threesomes and grown men cavorting in diapers that the final frontier of kinkiness is to opt out altogether. There's also the fact that I've just revealed my vow while thoroughly entwined with him. What are the ethics of that?

But despite the laugh, we have at last begun having the conversation that has been hanging over us, and it doesn't go at all as I'd expected. One of my quest's prompts was Jake's telling me that he didn't love me. It wasn't just what he said, either, but the way he said it, his tone a mix of surprise—what a strange notion; how could I ever have thought as much?—and preemptive self-righteousness. That we're talking right now rather than casting off clothes on our

way to the bedroom is in part due to his having made me so doubtful of my own responses. I couldn't believe that he was able to feel
what I felt and not acknowledge an additional something—something spiritual, almost. The alternative was that he simply hadn't
felt it, whatever he and his body told me. It was unnerving to think
that in those most intimate moments, I'd been alone in my feelings.
It scared me off a little, I suppose. And maybe that's what makes
good sex so unraveling—it takes you places where you're completely
on your own and where any sense of self is obliterated, a place beyond language, a place that's almost impossible to describe afterward, like a kind of alien abduction. (Alien abduction? I know—but
that's what good sex will do.)

Now Jake is telling me that I was right to have quizzed him so
intensely about it, that it had taken my absence to make him think
about what I'd asked him and to question what he'd told me. My
return, he says, has made him feel that, yes, this really is something
that might not ebb like other infatuations, something that can't be
found in another's kiss (yes, he's been doing some searching of his
own these past few months). Going on, he explains that he'd always
assumed we wouldn't be compatible in everyday life, that we
wouldn't get along on some level, though he's not sure why he ever
thought that. Finally, he comes round to the subject of his ghostly
girlfriend.

They are still together. Sort of. He still believes the relationship
is over, yet he still hasn't done anything to officially end it.

"Want to know the really ironic thing?" he asks, and I'm not sure
if I do. "I've made love to you more often than to my girlfriend lately.
We haven't had sex in eighteen months."

He next asks if it's all right to kiss me, and what can I say? It's
precious, the kiss that follows, salted somehow by all the tears that

I've shed over him in the past. And from amid our tangled, unchaste mess, I hear him say this, softly, as if daring himself: "I love you a bit, I think." It may sound like a measly half-measure to you, but I am so in thrall to this moment, it's like gold, and I cling to it as we cling to each other. Later, he kneels before me, leaning this way and that, trying to see me from every angle, just like he used to. "So where does this take us?" he asks. "Marriage and babies?"

It's something I've heard him say before, only in a brasher, more jokey voice. As he sees it—or, at least, as he *saw* it—this electric connection we share is simply a sign of powerful biological compatibility—nature goading us on to go forth and multiply. This explanation has enabled him to obey (with contraception, that is) what his body is telling him without having to trouble his evolved mind. He felt what I felt, it's just that he categorized those feelings as physical, whereas for me they felt physical, emotional, spiritual, intellectual, even. I was incapable of experiencing them as something polarized.

Women see and feel things more holistically, Shere Hite says in *Women and Love*. She goes on to suggest that rather than being rooted in repression, women's widespread inability to split mind from body, love from sex, harks back to a pre–Garden of Eden rite in which sex carried spiritual and religious meaning and was worshipped as the key to rebirth.

The separation of body and mind is a Western tradition. The Kama Sutra, for instance, though regarded today as nothing more than an encyclopedia of positions, emphasizes the role of the mind in good sex. Sheikh Nafzawi's *The Perfumed Garden*, written in fourteenth-century Tunis and dismissed by colonials as smut, likewise dwelt on the parts that the mind and the soul must play in meaningful sex.

In recent decades, science has taken up the baton from religion and philosophy and deepened the mind-body divide. In particular, it has demystified the metaphysics of sexual allure. Scientists tell us that if a woman hugs a man for more than a few minutes, she will necessarily start to grow attached. So-called sexperts have done their bit, too. In showing that sex is something that can be studied and improved upon, they have turned us all into Don Juans. Writing almost 150 years ago, the Goncourt brothers noted that "man is betrayed, not served, by his organs." As they had learned in the ballrooms and brothels of belle epoque Paris, "Touch this or that switch in a woman and out comes either pleasure or truth: you can make her admit at will that she is having an orgasm or that she loves you. This is appalling." And what's to say that some of those women weren't faking their raptures? That truly would have appalled them.

Back at Jake's, denied our usual resolution—the one we're so good at together—we reach a place we've never made it to before. We sit companionably together while he calls that uncle from out of town—the one who might have derailed our lunch, the one who wasn't a made-up excuse after all. We look up restaurants for their dinner together, and find one close to my place, so he can drop me off. It's dark outside now, and I tell him that in the past, those drives back across the ragged bits of London that separate us had always been tinged with bleakness for me. We'd never talk much. My hand would be resting on his knee and he'd sometimes turn to kiss me at red lights, but mentally we were already edging back into our very separate lives. Each junction that we passed represented another failure to communicate all that I had to say. I was oppressed by the sense that there was a question I should ask him, one that would make him open up to me and tell me where we were really headed—tell me what I wanted to hear.

This time, the streets are the same but everything else is different.

It's as if by merely naming that tense melancholy, we've robbed it of some of its hold over us. "I know what you mean," he says, and the sense of being understood is almost as good as "I love you a bit, I think." Maybe that was what I needed to hear all along. "Thank you for taking my hand," he says when we pull up outside my house. "I thought it was a lunch to show we were through," he adds. Yes, I think, so did I.

Later on that evening, he texts to tell me to look outside. In the sharp, starry night, a shadow is edging across the moon, and from our separate lives, we watch the eclipse together.

Standing at my darkened window, phone in hand, I think about what Jake told me earlier, about the deep irony of the fact that while I've been trying to understand his way of thinking, he's been coming around to mine. It seems sad that we've grown to mistrust some of our most profound experiences. For all that we elevate intercourse as an athletic art form, as something to perfect and improve on, to introduce gadgets to and to talk about—to talk through (just when did sex become so *chatty*?)—we have ceased to believe in its mystery. Perhaps it's because after feeling similar passion in the embraces of three, four or forty different people, it becomes hard not to depersonalize it, not to notch up those shivery thrills as mere biology, as our body responding the way a body will. And yet those feelings play a crucial role in love. Once you've unplugged their connection to your heart, how easy is it to reconnect them when you finally settle down? I've been desperately trying to keep the faith, I now realize, clinging to the idea that sex is never *just* sex.

The quest for oneness is key to the romantic urge. It *is* the romantic urge, Aristophanes argued in Plato's *Symposium*. We make it vivid in its sexual manifestation, as we squish our bodies together, burrowing into each other in a search for unity. We lock gazes, tongues, limbs. In public, we will often try to maintain that oneness, with gentle gestures like an arm thrown over the back of a chair or knees inclined toward each other.

With Jake, physical unity had felt so profound, I was unmoored without the concomitant psychological bond. I needed us to exist in a sphere beyond the increasingly nocturnal, silent world of bodily intensities that we'd created for ourselves. Those experiences were so vivid, yet they seemed unreal without any significant spillover into waking hours, only those wordless drives from his flat back to mine. We may appear to have tamed sex through giggly mockery— through the whips and rubber corsets in sex-shop windows—or through numbing overexposure, yet when it comes to the hard stuff, a wildness remains.

Intellectual, emotional nearness needs to be nurtured with time and care. Sex always stopped us in our conversational tracks. It made anything we tried to say seem trivial by comparison; it short-circuited friendship. Then again, sex engendered its own camaraderie, and it's this that Jake and I have both underestimated. Seeing him again after all these months, I realize that an approximate kinship has built up without our being aware of it. Beneath all those torrid feelings lay another, less fickle emotion: fondness.

And yet, despite my vow, my instinctive response to Jake remains breathtakingly physical. Even his texts arrive with a sock to my heart, sending my mood swinging one way or the other depending on tone and content. I don't use the word *heart* in the cute sense of candy and teddy bears, either: I mean it at its most literal and bloodily pounding.

I see him occasionally over the coming weeks. Jake is the ultimate test and the temptation is nearly too much, yet the push-pull of my vow makes resistance almost pleasurable. It's a kind of power I've attained, and I'm relishing it. It makes me wonder, too: if I'd stood by my initial decision to not sleep with Jake until he'd formalized his breakup, would he have stood by me?

It's a difficult task, winding back a relationship, but my commitment to my vow gives me a chance to see how things might have panned out with Jake had I insisted on a sign of commitment before sleeping with him. His flat has grown to represent a kind of erotic playground for me—an impression fortified by its basement position and open-plan layout—so I suggest activities that keep us away. "Want to see a film?" I text. He has too much work, and a stormy cloud edges over my afternoon.

"Text back and let him know what he's missing," my sister says, laughing. But for once, I'm in the mood to listen. It's humiliating to be obsessing over texts like a fifteen-year-old, but because that's what I'm doing, I want guidance, I want specific instructions—I want my reply dictated to me word for word. My sister looks alarmed: the penalties for bad romantic advice are steep. "I don't know," she says, shrugging. "Just say 'shame, dot dot dot.'" She is a great one for ellipses, my sister, and it strikes me that this might be her secret. It suggests mystery, something she's keeping to herself, and it drives her admirers mad. She picks but she never pursues— the running is always theirs. Her newest catch might not be such a catch, though—a wild-haired artist who sells sarongs in a market stall to pay his rent.

It's getting late by the time I do as my sister tells me, and it's later still by the time Jake's reply arrives. He hadn't declined, he protests, he'd love to see me. "What are you doing right now?"

It worked. Or did it? Within the hour, I'm slipping out of the house and into his waiting car. It's gone midnight and the clocks have just edged forward, robbing us of an hour, though the mist-drenched air makes it seem more like autumn than the start of summertime. As we coast through sleeping streets, I repeat Jake's question in my head: what am I doing?

Here's what I've told myself: we'll hang out and chat about French cinema, perhaps watch a DVD in lieu of the film we didn't see earlier on. I'm fooling no one, of course—not myself and least of all Jake, whose hands venture beneath my sweater to find lace and silk. My cover blown, I give up on conversation and let my tongue do a different kind of talking. Is it fair on Jake to do this—to go so far and then stop? I fall asleep apologizing, with Jake curled around my back, his face on my neck. Maybe half an hour later I wake to the best kiss I've ever tasted. Befuddled by sleep and hormones and, yes, love—or something that feels confusingly similar—I very nearly give in. For a fleeting second I feel a ripple of force and think that maybe I'll give in to avoid its becoming something else, but then I return to my senses: I remember the tears and the hurt and the claustrophobic feeling of being trapped forever in the same plot. I remember my vow.

The tussle between us—between him, me and myself—is over in two, maybe three seconds. In the wakeful quiet that follows, listening to Jake's breathing as it slows and then deepens back into sleep, I think about what just happened. I resisted, he resisted, and yet I don't feel good about it. I feel inept, and it occurs to me that going all the way might be the lazy girl's option. Without that to offer, my arsenal of tricks is as skimpy as a thong. At the back of my mind is a thought that seems like a leftover from some teen novel, the thought that if such sentiments of unworthiness and ineptitude are lurking in my heart, it's because I'm not feeling loved enough.

Over the past few weeks, a small pile of books has been growing by my bedside. It's made up not of the usual novels but of books about chastity. I'd thought they might offer me some tips on how to cope with temptation or the loneliness that can take over in its absence. Now I'm not so sure. One volume recommends hugging your friends extra long, another gazing lovingly at yourself in the mirror each morning. Begin each day with a meditative breathing exercise, suggests a third. Or what about reaching for your apron and having fun in the kitchen? "Bake cookies, brownies, muffins. Ask your girlfriends for assistance. Guys will do anything for homemade baked goods," writes Pulitzer Prize–winning *Washington Post* reporter Laura Sessions Stepp in her book *Unhooked: How Young Women Pursue Sex, Delay Love and Lose at Both*. Well, I could bake Jake some cookies, but he's far too metrosexual to thank me for all that fatty sugar. Could I make dinner? I could not. The best I could manage would be to "assemble" dinner and hide the packaging. We women have been let off knowing how to cook or darn a sock, but we're expected to have other skills. As David Kepesh, the sexagenarian narrator of Philip Roth's novella *The Dying Animal,* so approvingly observes: "The decades since the Sixties have done a remarkable job of completing the sexual revolution. This is a generation of astonishing fellators." Is it surprising that when a girl I know found herself dumped for the third time in a year, she enrolled in fellatio classes?

But I generalize. My sister has cooked for her long-haired friend. I came back late one evening to find the house fragranced with spiced meat and sweet couscous, the two of them chatting conspiratorially in the kitchen. She's also visited him at the market, bearing festive cookies. Another time, he brought his guitar over and I heard them singing duets together.

The next day, Jake and I lie on the sofa together while Sunday ambles by, birdsong blending with the random selection of tunes playing on his laptop. There are songs that remind me that he's a decade older; fragments of film scores that hint at fragments of story lines; and then this refrain: "I love you," its singer singing those three words as easily as the blackbird trilling outside. On the table with our teacups and crumby plates, Jake's name is joined with his absentee girlfriend's on a bill. There's something else, too, a flyer for a film with a one-word title: *Liar*.

Real life is rarely as subtle as fiction. Later, it will occur to me that while I'd been searching for understated, elegant truths, a starker wisdom was staring at me all along. But not just yet. Because for now, the intimacy Jake and I have created in the absence of full sex is almost more intoxicating. Early-morning kisses, the simple delight of waking beside him, before I'm alert enough to start looking for hidden meanings—these beat any postcoital glow. To properly sleep with someone—to draw warmth from the same blanket and greet the next day together—weaves its own spell, I realize. This is the intimacy that was missing from my twenties.

Very quickly, things between us assume an all-too-familiar pattern. One night, I'm up late to do a radio phone-in show and divert my cab back from the studio to Jake's—at four in the morning. He greets me with a kiss so good that I feel like I'm cheating on my vow right there in the doorway. Dawn finds me lying in his arms bathed in the whiteness of his bedroom, a parody of purification. The strengthening light cuts silhouettes on the shades—clear, simple. Why am I really resisting? I wonder. Wasn't my vow in some way a direct response to Jake? Well, here I am, so why not just give in to the deliciousness of it all and give up on the vow?

The real challenge comes a few nights later. I find myself at a party right around the corner from Jake's and can't resist texting in case he's home. The possibility of a reply adds a frisson to the evening. It's on my mind later as I chat with Megan, a colleague's exgirlfriend. Our host is generous and everyone in the room has a champagne sheen, but not Megan; hers is all natural. It must be two years since we last ran into each other, and I'm struck by the change in her. She radiates the kind of centered calm that seems like a New Age myth until you see it. She's still single, she tells me, and is focusing on her work and her children. What she doesn't reveal until I bump into her again, months later, is that she is actually in the middle of her own year of celibacy.

Jake does text back, and it's only when he lets me in that I notice how tipsy I am, and how unusual this is in his teetotal company. Taking my coat, he takes in my party clothes, and I realize that I'm dressed as a person he's rarely glimpsed. There it is again—the separateness of our lives. It's as if another barrier has gone up between us, alongside my vow.

It's also thrilling, and what follows is the hottest, most X-rated nonsex I've ever had. Heck, it's hotter than sex, which makes it feel illegal to me, and raises the temperature still higher. Every atom of my being yearns for him, and the more I get of him, the more greedy it makes me. It's urgent and lingering, yielding and resisting, probing and caressing—a feverish, soft-hard coil of contradictions that tightens around us, since we cannot follow it to its natural conclusion. It's wholly physical and yet beyond physical, since we dissolved into each other when he pressed me up against the wall and pinned my arms above my head; when he bit the nape of my neck while dipping his hand; when he slid down my trembling, lust-drunk body to his knees. It's also a kind of torture, made tougher still by the fact that Jake is someone I've already slept with. Knowing in graphic detail what I'm resisting makes it almost impossible to do so—especially when he whispers again that he might be falling a little in love with me. Leaning back to look at him, I notice that there's a tear in his eye, and suddenly it's too much for me—I can't help myself. Oh, my chastity remains intact, but instead of yielding my body I give up my heart. I match his feelings and raise them, telling him that I'm falling for him more than a little bit.

TEN

April... in London

Abstainer, n: A weak person who yields to the temptation of denying himself a pleasure.

—Ambrose Bierce, *The Devil's Dictionary*

When I signed up to this year, I couldn't resist thinking of all the things I'd have the time and energy for without sex and its breathless pursuit to occupy my spare hours. I'd write a novel! The creative energy I sank into imagining what such-and-such a guy might be thinking—well, I'd put it to good use. And instead of taking fellatio classes, I'd wrap my tongue around a new language—Italian, why not? Pilates was another. I would become one of those glowing Amazonians whose no-makeup look really is natural, the kind who can get away with wearing their workout leggings outside the gym.

Leaving aside the novel writing and the Italian (I certainly have), I've averaged a single Pilates class every other week or three. It's not that I haven't felt motivated: I have, sometimes. No, my problem with Pilates is that it seems so me-me-me-ish. It feels like part of that cult of perfection and self-obsession that keeps us away from one another on a deeper level. Strive tirelessly for a body that's a temple, and you'll worship at it. That was my excuse, anyway.

Pilates is based partly on yoga, and yoga, as we often forget, is part of a complex Hindu philosophical tradition. The hard bit isn't standing on your head or firming your gluteus maximus, it's using your head to attain a higher state of consciousness. Chastity also has a tradition, a tradition that my quest goes ironically against: in its religious context, it is all about transcending not only the body but the self as well.

In *The Cult of the Born-Again Virgin,* Wendy Keller offers a step-by-step guide to staying chaste until the right man comes along. One of her program's key props is an index card on which followers list the twenty things they most like about themselves. "Put this into your jewelry box because it's the most precious adornment you own. Read it aloud every time you open the box. Repeat it every day. Make another copy and keep it in your purse. Heck, repeat it a hundred times a day if you want really rapid results," she schools. Ask me to empty out the contents of my bag, and you'll find no such card, but the accompanying introspection can be hard to avoid.

This morning, of course, I did actually make it to that Pilates class. While my body is in no danger of being mistaken for a temple, strolling home, I do notice that I'm inhabiting it in a way that it's easy to forget is possible if you lead a sedentary, desk-bound lifestyle that doesn't include treadmills or clubbing—or sex. It's a pretty day—blue sky above, green park off to one side, the cherry blossom pink beneath my feet. Couples stroll by draped about each other like garments, and the cafés are full, each table orbited by a dog or a child's scooter. I'm struck again by the oddness of this second act between me and Jake—how its time frame fits so snugly with the first. Not only the season but also the geography seems to match: here is the exact place where I sat in the sunshine, texting him "happy birthday."

For the first time, there's parity in our relationship. I want more of him than he's able to give emotionally; he wants more of me than I'm prepared to yield physically. This should be more consoling than it feels. As it is, I've been plotting each date in my diary, desperately hoping they'll join up to form a coherent, continuous whole. They do not. Truthfully, these are not so much dates as assignations. Though each time I manage to return to my chaste senses on the very brink of breaking my vow, our encounters invariably take place at night, following on from preludes that are increasingly wordless. There is none of the charged sparring of Hepburn and Tracy here, though when we do chat, conversation gravitates to film plots. Jake has begun using them to explain his feelings about us, and on the days when I don't see him, I hunt for DVDs. Sitting alone in the dark, I watch his ideas about us play out, hungry for clues. Most of the films are French, none is contemporary and few end happily. He is fictionalizing us, I realize. We may be classic but we're also over, trapped in a past-tense palette of black and white or saturated sixties color like bugs in amber.

Meanwhile, every minute that I spend with Jake risks making a mockery of my chaste rules. Have I been cheating? According to the letter of my vow, I haven't, not quite, though in spirit I've probably racked up enough transgressions to have me expelled from any chaste academy. Would I have been a harsher lawmaker had I known that he would step back into my life? I'm not sure—it might have made things easier, but then surely that would also make it wrong. For his part, Jake insists that I need him, that in order to validate my vow, I have to confront credible temptation. Female sexuality has long been defined by the male gaze. Even Anaïs Nin, the author of legendarily saucy stories and journals, once confessed, "Flirting with other men, not writing, helped me to become a woman." (It's worth noting that she also described herself as a "winged doormat.") Was it the same with its opposite—did I really need to rebuff a man's advances in order to feel chaste?

I'd thought that my vow was an act of personal rebellion against what had felt like a masculine relationship code, one that cajoled me into denying what my own body was telling me, but perhaps my very definition of *sex* is part of the same problem. I mean, is it really all about penetration? Wasn't I being a bit phallocentric?

Magazine articles may encourage us to think of low-commitment sex as liberating, but many women who lived through the sixties would argue differently. In her memoir *Making Trouble,* Lynne Segal, who spent the 1970s in the thick of the second-wave feminist movement, describes the disappointments from which it sprang. "As many of my friends reminded me, it was the lack of ecstasy, or even real intimacy, in sexual engagement with men in the Sixties that first inspired them to talk of their own 'liberation' . . . Some women had experienced both the orgasms and the intimacy so publicly celebrated in the 'Summer of Love' of 1967. Nevertheless, few felt free from sexual doubts and conflict in their relationships with men." Feminist discourse soon turned on the "myth of the vaginal orgasm" as the cause of their feelings of failure and dissatisfaction, and she recalls later meeting men in relationships with radical feminists who flat-out refused to engage in penetrative sex, claiming it was intrinsically "anti-feminist." (Perhaps I should put that to Jake?) Others became "political lesbians," and gradually, the movement's many splinter groups fell to bickering among themselves. These days, it's hard to find a woman who'll hold up her hand to be counted a feminist.

And what of the movement's triumphs? In a new millennium, the depiction of sex still seems filtered through the male gaze. It can be hard to tell a women's magazine from a men's by looking at the pictures alone—photo shoots aimed at selling clothes to women are strikingly similar to those selling women to men. As Ariel Levy asserted in her Zeitgeist-pipping *Female Chauvinist Pigs,* "A tawdry, cartoonlike version of female sexuality has become so ubiquitous, it no longer seems particular. What we once regarded as a *kind* of sexual expression we now view *as* sexual expression."

I daresay Freud would have had views on my quest, too. Miss A, the in-denial nymphomaniac? I mention this having lately discovered that twelve months is the "drying-out" period recommended by Sex Addicts Anonymous. Their Web site lists qualifying traits, and some of them seem troublingly applicable. "Has your sexual or romantic behavior ever left you feeling hopeless, alienated from others, or suicidal?" for instance. Thankfully not the last, but hopeless and alienated? For sure. And what about this: "Does each new relationship continue to have the same destructive patterns which prompted you to leave the last relationship?" If it's also allowed that they leave you, then yes. Yes! This thing with Jake is the *Groundhog Day* of relationships.

But the most pressing question on my mind right now is this: have I spared myself any pain in not going all the way this time round? It may not seem a fair test, given that Jake and I did sleep together prevow (if we hadn't, would I have been able to resist seeing sex as the solution right now?), but I have to admit that, yes, holding out *has* made a difference. I almost wish it weren't so—Erma Franklin makes capitulation sound so sweet.

The very act of pondering all this wins me back a bit more perspective. Rather than getting sad or mad or simply dissolving into a salty puddle, I'm able to appreciate, for instance, that this relationship is bad not only for me but for Jake, too. Without its distraction, he'd have to work through the situation with the woman he continues to call his girlfriend despite claiming not to have seen her in months or slept with her in still longer.

I feel uncomfortably close to this other woman I've never met; we each have half of the same relationship. In a tug of war, who would win, I wonder, the cerebral or the physical? Because ironically, my vow of chastity seems to be making things with Jake even more physical: the line I've drawn has become a titillating challenge, a boundary to be breached. It reintroduces the tantalizing notion of trespass, of the forbidden. Just as the chastity belt—never widespread, but in its time a tortuous way for men to own women's sexuality—has become kinky, so my vow has become tremblingly erotic.

The corrupt and corrupting cad the Vicomte de Valmont discovered as much in Pierre Choderlos de Laclos's *Les Liaisons Dangereuses*. Initially, Madame de Tourvel's pious virtue merely goads him on to destroy her, but gradually he falls under its spell. "I thought my heart withered up and, finding I had nothing left but my senses, I pitied myself for a premature old age. Madame de Tourvel has given me back the charming illusions of youth," he writes to his old flame, the scheming Marquise de Merteuil.

It's been ten days since I was last in touch with Jake, and the realization that I'm counting is dismaying. Passing the café from where I sent him last year's birthday text, the one that finally set me on this chaste path, I remember how determined I was back then to seize control of my emotional life. This in turn causes me to act in a way that is briskly out of character. I tap out another text to Jake, this one a short, simple request that we meet for a drink. He replies an instant later—yes, just let him know where and when.

I'm actually following some very specific advice from Nina, who has been insisting that I call a summit with him. My chosen location is the bar of a restaurant, a sleekly classic place with booths and an Edward Hopper–ish vibe, its menu yearning for New York, its skyscraper prices very definitely belonging to London. Outside, it's the start of a bank holiday weekend and the first fine evening of the year. Inside, plush Sinatra songs recall Christmas and log fires. Why did I pick this place? Everything about it indicates distance, phoniness.

Straight to the point, Nina had warned, but what was my point? If she were sitting here, she'd have a bullet-pointed treaty drawn up and ready to sign. Me, I've nothing. A glass of white wine isn't helping—its coolness belongs to the airy evening beyond rather than this fuggy interior, and each sip dilutes my resolution. The man sitting opposite me may as well be a stranger. He is silent, his manner a faultless mix of the wounded and the defensive.

"I had things I needed to say," I begin, and then skitter to a halt.

"I thought you might," he replies, dropping his gaze.

The table feels huge and I feel lost. Even as I'd rehearsed them in my head, the things I wanted to say sounded hollow. Now they seem so obvious that I can't bring myself to utter them. He isn't ready for another relationship, that much is dazzlingly clear. He is hunkered down over there on his side of the table, using the husk of his past relationship as a shield lest the menu prove too flimsy. Why tell him things he has known all along? It's me who needs the talking to: "Hephzibah, you fool. Even if he wanted to, he can't give you what you want just now. And guess what? He doesn't want to." Maybe this is what Nina was getting at with her summit idea—maybe she was just too kind-hearted to tell me these things herself.

Across the table, Jake seems to sense that the crisis has passed.

He orders a salad and tucks in. I order a second glass of wine and wish I hadn't. The restaurant is full by the time we leave, heading out onto streets drenched in holiday quiet with a film in mind, maybe another bar. Crossing an eerily deserted Piccadilly, we stray into Green Park and find it wrapped in the kind of darkness that's unexpected in the city, broken only by faux-historic streetlamps beneath which lost tourists and other couples wander. A tramp passes by, chatting animatedly to himself, and I—who am after all having a relationship with my own self—smile through the night at him, one deluded soul to another.

Jake kisses me, and then he takes my hand and leads me back to his car, wordlessly navigating us out of the center, toward his place. "That was decisive," I say, and he puts a finger to his lips. They are the only words either of us will speak for hours. Later, drifting in and out of sleep, I am fitfully aware of farcically failing to have our conversation. Perhaps it's something easier done in the dark, I think—the world outside seems simplified by night, its lines neat and crisp. But then somehow my eyes close again.

In waking hours, when I'm totting up Jake's negatives, the fact that he's begun keeping a dream journal is right up there. There's something so melancholic about it, the way he begins each day chasing the unreachable, a world that recedes with each word he pins down. I don't know what he writes the next morning, but I remember a strange, fragmentary dream, in which I get up and head into Soho, leaving Jake sleeping. It's weekend Soho, very different from its weekday self, and I get stuck amid the boozed-up hurly-burly, unable to reach him by phone, my heart pounding with inexplicable anxiety.

It seems to me that I was perhaps enacting what I'd been unable to do—present my ultimatum and then walk away—glossing it with excuses for my failure. I really had intended to tell Jake what I should have told him months earlier, to call me if ever he found himself free and desiring of another relationship. The dream seemed to suggest that I feared giving up on the notion of an "us" would signal a return to the chaos of my twenties—a version of that messy Soho scene. Except that now I have my vow, and no more excuses.

At some point during that long, tangled night, we did talk, but we talked about sex, not emotions. We talked about what my vow stops us from doing; we didn't broach the subject of what his situation stops him from giving. How is it that I can be so free with this man in bed, and yet feel so anxious around him the rest of the time? What we talk about when we talk about sex are the mechanics; emotional intimacy is infinitely harder to discuss.

In the UK, which has the highest rate of teenage pregnancy in western Europe, children receive sex education at an ever younger age, but it is only the physiological aspects that are compulsory. Teachers are under no obligation to brief pupils on the emotional dimension.

One of the gentler revelations of my vow is how it has made me feel things that I lack a current vocabulary for. The words that I find myself reaching for need dusting off. They carry a mothball tang and evoke the ghostly rustle of crinolines. Before I embarked upon this year, these words would have seemed corsetcd—unyielding, inexpressive. Yet their antiquation leaves scope for personalization— it's what makes them so versatile. *Yearning, forbearance, adoration*—I can now appreciate the roiling depths beneath their prim surface, and I've remembered that *romance* is also a verb.

The next morning, Jake makes tea, and, sitting at the breakfast bar, we finally begin to have the conversation I'd intended to have in that other bar, some eighteen hours earlier. What makes it easier is that I can now use a different tense. It's become "what I was going to tell you" and "what I should have said"—conditional and safely contained within the past.

Unfortunately, Jake's response is future tense. Last night, I'd been going to tell him things he already knew; now he is telling me stuff I already know. He's a coward about getting out of relationships, he says, but even if he finalized the breakup with his girlfriend, he wouldn't come immediately round on bended knee. It's an odd choice of phrase, but, then, my vow seems to have flooded everything with sepia. He adds that he has thought about it—about whether we two could be more. He's told a friend about me and I've been declared perfect, but still, Jake doubts we'd have enough in common. And there are his past failures—he doesn't trust himself not to get it wrong again.

The saddest thing about moments like these is that their scripts are so clichéd. Our hurt isn't fully our own. We are doomed to cause each other pain in the same old ways. Yet even in my chaste state, it seems wrong to resist the sheer physical rightness of us. Our fit feels a truth that trumps any other—and I'm not just talking about sex. We share space seamlessly, moving around each other like water or air. There seems an elemental rightness to us, so much so that it feels out of our hands—and ultimately, isn't that what we're all after in love? We still flinch at the idea of choosing, hoping that a chubby-thighed Cupid will glance us with one of his arrows and make the decision for us.

Jake agrees when I suggest that it would be wrong not to find out whether there is more between us, but this small victory feels forced, as if he's let me wangle it so he can duck out of a conversation that he wishes had ended a while ago. We'll spend time together less intensely, we decide. More daylight hours. "Is this allowed?" he asks, leaning in to kiss me.

So there it is; the upshot of all that anxious thought and chat is that we end up making out in one of the few spots of his apartment where we've not done so before. I once read a short story about a futuristic forensic device that could be beamed around a room to reveal not blood but lust. If we'd had such a gadget, Jake's apartment would have been awash with electric blue.

Back at our local café, Nina takes one look at me before thrusting Alfie at her husband and switching her smoothie to a stronger order.

Together we overanalyze my situation, pooling our own anecdotes with those of friends and friends' friends. Between sips, we pore over incidents and instances, feeling our way toward some great Theory of Jake.

Do men indulge in these storytelling rituals? The narratives that we weave from these scraps of stories—the giddy beginnings and vague endings, the missing middles—sometimes end up being more real than the relationships themselves. The sex is real, but the rest? The rest is what we decide to make of it, how we spin it over cocktails with the girls. After one supersized glass of wine—call it a half-bottle—it occurs to me that Jake and I might actually have broken up, if it's possible to break something that doesn't wholly exist. Listening to my story, it would definitely seem that way.

Relationship advice is more therapeutic than practical. We lay out the problem and clutch eagerly at our friends' suggestions, longing to believe that they hold the solution. Yet how often do we follow it through? In the context of the relationship, those friendly words of sound counsel rarely seem such a good fit.

Transposing lessons learned from our own relationships is tricky enough: we need to believe that it's possible—that the sad situations in which we find ourselves again and again will somehow prove beneficial—but at the same time, a part of us doggedly resists the notion that love can be schemed for.

And then there's the fact that so many of romance's game plans date back to a time when the rules were very different, when sex was a rapture not arrived at quite so easily and its implications were ineluctably long-term—a lifetime of domesticity blissful or fractious, or else the ignominy of rumor. Pregnancy was harder to avoid and more dangerous whether gone through with or not.

When Jake first blew back into my life, withholding full sex was empowering. Now it has become its own titillating end. Perversely, I can sense that it's made Jake feel licensed to drift along in the same casual way.

The next day I feel surprisingly fine about it all, though midmorning finds me tidying and upping the volume on some too-chirpy music—bad signs both. I'm meant to be having tea with Rafiq and it's tempting to cancel but I force myself out of the house.

We meet in a pastry shop that closes early, though not before Rafiq has insisted I sample an orgy of sugary delights. Chased back out onto empty streets, we head toward his car, where my business cards—I've accepted some freelance work from him and their delivery is the real reason for our meeting—are stowed in the trunk. As we pass another cake shop, this one still open, Rafiq ducks in to buy more dainty confections to go. Standing in line, he tries to tempt me. "What about that one? There, with the coffee icing and vanilla center?" Rafiq is Muslim, and while he isn't religious enough to not drink, he doesn't drink much. Perhaps he's trying to get me tipsy on sugar.

Dr. John Harvey Kellogg, the cornflake king who didn't allow even his honeymoon to compromise a lifelong devotion to chastity, railed about sex in a series of publications. Intercourse, he declared, could "retard growth, weaken the constitution and dwarf the intellect."

Tobacco, alcohol, corsets and constipation were all hazardous to the chaste, whose resolve could also be weakened by overheated rooms and too much time spent sitting down. Oh, and waltzing. Cake was not quite up there with porn, but, along with jellies and "fine-flour breadstuffs," it was potent enough, Kellogg cautioned, to have been the undoing of clergymen making their parish rounds.

Back at his car, Rafiq reaches for his jacket and pulls my cards from the pocket like a magician. Handing the box to me, he simultaneously opens the door on the passenger side. "Do you have plans?" he asks. "Because I was just going to hang out in the garden, watch a bit of cricket—eat cake. You could join me."

There's something missing from the invitation, though I can't decide what, and I'm so keen to be distracted from mooning over Jake that I don't really care. The garden belongs to his friend Raj, whom I met back at the singles party. Rafiq is house-sitting, and as we drift into tonier zip codes, the light changes. The buildings here are a dazzling white, and tall, too, as if they know that the sky is theirs to reach for. A bulky burglar alarm blinks prominently on each, guarding a shuttered calm. Inside, Raj's place is immaculate— the kind of immaculate that tells you to slip off your shoes, which I do before following a stairway down to an open-plan basement that backs onto the garden. The house is rented, Rafiq explains. Entirely rented. The cutlery and crockery, sheets and towels, even the supposedly personal touches like the misshapen vase and the brightly spattered canvas—all are rented. The only items here that belong to Raj are a few stacks of paperwork and some clothing.

Something about all this plush cream carpet makes me feel like an intruder, and I realize I'm tiptoeing. Tiptoeing into the kitchen where Rafiq is making tea, tiptoeing out into the garden where he has set out more cakes—more sugary, chocolaty goo, melting slightly in the afternoon sun. He plies me with pastries; I try to resist. There is a battle going on between us, and it isn't entirely about choux puffs.

When the sun vanishes behind a cloud, we move back inside and I hover over the sofa while Rafiq fusses in the kitchen. To take the chair is unfriendly, but to sit on the sofa? The far end seems presumptuous—Rafiq couldn't then take the chair; I'd be forcing him onto the sofa and I don't know that that's where I want him. The middle is tempting, but it's the end nearest the chair that wins. That way, he can walk around the coffee table and take the other end or he can opt for the chair. He opts for the chair, and I find I'm relieved, though it does nothing to ease a growing awkwardness, especially because the chair seems somehow farther away with someone sitting in it.

We're already running out of chat, but there is something hypnotic about the lulls. They feel elastic, like they could stretch and stretch. Just then, an enormous flat-screen TV leaps to life and the room is filled with the sound of leather on willow, a polite ripple of applause. I feel like joining in—a distraction! These cricket updates are the only alleviation in what turns out to be six long hours of awkwardness.

Early on it was established that he would drive me home on the way back to his place, so to call myself a cab would appear rude. After a couple of hours, I run out of questions and begin saying anything that pops into my head. He responds, or doesn't. At no point could it be said that we are engaged in actual conversation. What am I doing here? What are we doing here? The plan was to catch up over tea and

collect those business cards. We've since drifted so far into unsched-
uled time that I worry that one of us should have left a trail of
crumbs—cake crumbs. When it's finally time to leave, Rafiq runs
upstairs and returns carrying my shoes. Just like on the night we met,
I feel like I've strayed into a scrambled version of *Cinderella*.

In its way, that epic Sunday afternoon spent sitting on the tan
leather rental couch proves more enlightening than hours and hours
on another kind of couch. I was waiting for something to happen.
I'd gone along out of curiosity, hardly stopping to ask myself what
might happen, what I might *like* to happen. The story seemed too
irresistible—a tall, dark, sad-eyed companion, a sunny afternoon
and an open-top sports car. I didn't really belong in it, I knew that,
but I couldn't resist seeing what it might be like if I did. As the re-
lentlessly solipsistic Nin put it, "Women see themselves as in a mirror in the eyes of the men who love them. I have seen in each man a
different woman—and a different life." The thing is, Rafiq wasn't
exactly in his own life that afternoon, either. In fact, it wasn't even
Raj's, not really. It was a hired backdrop—tasteful, desolate. But
perhaps Rafiq really had intended to eat cake and watch the cricket.
Maybe I was reading erotic intent into an innocent invitation whose
only unchaste aspirations lay in the pastry box. Could it be that
chastity is turning me into Anaïs Nin? Of all the conversations we
could have had and didn't, one about faith—about the nature of his
beliefs—might have answered these questions I'm left with. It didn't
occur to me to bring it up at the time—it seemed too personal.

The afternoon also forces me to acknowledge that aside from a
few debatably aimed social kisses that somehow landed on lips
rather than cheeks, I have never been much of a move maker. In this
respect, I conform to gender archetypes. Surveys consistently show
that men remain more likely to initiate sex than women. Not that

that has let us off the hook: historically, women have been held accountable for keeping men's libidos in check. Good wives, it was declared, went to bed in long flannel nightgowns.

I've been up since five A.M. trying and failing to complete an overdue article, and now I'm stuck in a minicab in hot sunshine. The morning rush hour is moving so slowly, time so quickly. I'm late, later. My destination is a big trade event on the other side of town, and I should have been there to meet one of my editors half an hour ago. When I finally make it to the press office, I'm handed a badge that I pin to my jacket while rushing off in the wrong direction. I'm so anxious to find my editor that when a text arrives I've read it before I can spot that it is from Jake. It's shifty-seeming—clearly sent so that he could say he'd sent it when he next ran into me, which he must have calculated would be soon.

Meanwhile, I'm later than late. Aiming for a shortcut, I take the stairs—backstage stairs, the kind conference-goers are not meant to see, fragrant with disinfectant. When I slip, the concrete is cruel, though humiliating rather than lethal. I bump to a halt a few feet down, my phone skittering behind me, just out of reach. Wincing, I glance down at my badge to see that there's a spelling mistake. I am Helpzibah. It also says I hail from Brussels, which feels fitting enough this morning.

Hours later, I'm standing chatting when suddenly Jake is there. He is wearing a shirt and jacket, looking as businesslike as I do. We are both other people today—other people who match each other. The knowing amusement on the face of the man I've been talking to says he knows a little of our history. We leave together, Jake and I, and it feels like a grand escape, stepping out into a day that has grown lovely while we've been stuck inside. Jake is being very proper, as if we really have just met, and over coffee, that distance remains. His gaze strays, fixes on passing women. His kiss good-bye is glancing. Afterward, I wander into a lingerie store and find myself contemplating an especially lacy line called Adored. Maybe men buy it for their girlfriends and wives, but it's likely that most of these bras and panties are bought by women precisely because they *don't* feel adored, because they feel their men's attention wandering. Cherished is another line, equally frilly and titillating. We make ourselves feel sexy to cheer ourselves up, and I'm no different. In the changing room I notice a lurid purple bruise blooming on my thigh.

I'm due at a work dinner in the same neighborhood, and with time to spare, I decide to take my bruised, sorry ass for a martini. My working day began at dawn, I reason, and it *is* cocktail hour. The bar is on the tenth floor, and in almost as many years of working in an office across the way, I've never been here. It is lovely. The evening's first glittering lights dot a pastel horizon, as the green park below darkens until only its paths and lakes are visible, glowing pale in the dusk.

The martini is working its magic, and at my feet is a bag of black lacy lingerie, but part of the thrill is being here alone. It will soon be time for me to leave and join my dinner crowd—a crowd convened, I should mention, by the Quiet Guy. (Remember him? We've been e-mailing ever since meeting back in October, and now work brings him to London.) Already, darkness has made a mirror of the window. Looking back at myself, I wonder: how did I get here?

A few evenings later, along comes the annual party that a year ago occasioned mine and Jake's first kiss. I regret going as soon as I step into its crammed din. The sound and heat are like extra dimensions in an already packed space. I stumble into the beery embrace of a group of friends and edge up to the mezzanine level with them. From there, I spot Jake arriving, cursorily scanning the room before vanishing behind a pillar. By the time I make it back down, he is deep in conversation with a blond Frenchwoman, his body angled toward her. A mutual friend spots me and nudges him, winning me a hello, a strictly social kiss, and an introduction to his companion. As she and I shake hands, he leans in to whisper something in her ear.

I feel precarious. I'm standing on the stairs in heels, but it isn't just that. When the Quiet Guy comes over to say hi, I am incredibly grateful for his height, for his clean good looks. Jake reveals another side of himself with the blonde, a side I rarely glimpse—slippery smooth and crafty. He looks tired, each and every one of those ten years that separate us etched on his face. But now his conversation is over, and he's stepping toward me, reaching for my hand. It's a gesture that betrays intimacy, and the Quiet Guy slips away, bound for the bar.

Jake lives just a short walk away and we leave together, squeezing by shoulders, catching hugs and dodging sloshes of beer. Later, when he kisses me, something happens that has never happened before: I find my thoughts drifting. Back along those cherry-lined, moonlit streets they go, back to the party, back to the Quiet Guy.

From Jake there is no acknowledgment that this marks the year since that first kiss, nor that this kind of assignation is precisely what we'd agreed to give up just a week earlier. We're putting ourselves back together when he picks up one of my shoes and holds it up, examining it. Another princess moment. Or perhaps not.

"Maybe I've made it too easy for you to say no," he says. However tamed sex seems, flirtation with desire's darker side is the commonest kind of fantasy. It's taken my assumed cloak of born-again virginity to bring it out in Jake.

Back home, I throw my dress and stockings into the laundry hamper. I don't know it, because the message gets lost in the ether, but the Quiet Guy BlackBerrys me about then, regretting that we hadn't chatted more and inviting me along to a play the following evening. In the morning, another e-mail goes the same way, but whereas I would have read all that I needed to know into the lack of response, the Quiet Guy—perhaps by definition a closer reader of silence—tries one last time, texting later that afternoon.

It's long and ultracontemporary. Three androgynous performers, a single chair set in the center of a bare stage and a pineapple as their only prop. Afterward, we wander off with the playwright in search of that elusive near-midnight last drink. Away from the theater, the evening acquires a serendipitous vibe, and suddenly a song from a Manhattan movie we all love comes on. Do we move from there to talking about New York, to talking about pancakes? I'm not keeping track, but it seems there is a diner in this city after all, out east and open twenty-four hours. I'm only moments from home, but somehow I find myself campaigning for a pancake pit stop across town, joining the Quiet Guy in cajoling along his friend.

London's answer to an all-night diner is as surreal as you'd imagine. We are seated in a horseshoe-shaped booth made of green leather. At some point, there is a sudden birthday announcement, and a waitress materializes with a slice of cake as an enormous screen plays a lurid happy-birthday video. The other customers look like juvenile drug dealers. Our table fills with fries, a full English breakfast for good measure and a stack of pancakes—the pancakes we failed to have in October. Rather than energize us, the food grounds us.

Sometime later, the Quiet Guy announces that he has no clear idea of when his flight home is the next day. "It's very unlike the way

I usually travel," he says. When our third member finally summons a cab, it doesn't really change anything. It's been the two of us right from the start, surreptitiously saving details about each other. He notices that we share a middle initial, I that we're the same age. We slither a little nearer along the green banquette on the pretext of him showing me the day's missing e-mails. Mine to him has done something odd, too: it has landed on his screen in red. There it is, so scarlet it may as well be throbbing.

Even with nowhere else to go, you can stay in a subterranean diner only so long, and eventually we haul ourselves up and out, our only plan being to go for a walk. It is still dark outside, though early birds are warming up for the dawn chorus. We are close to the city's old meat market and stop to get coffee-shop directions from a man in white wellies and a blood-spattered jacket. All around us, similarly dressed men toil in silence, chalky, industrious apparitions. Ferraris is just around the corner, a rare real workers' café that serves exactly what you need at this hour: instant coffee, milky and sweet.

Out on the street again, polystyrene cups in hands, we spot a garden square, moated by the swooping drive to an underground car park. It's locked, but, balancing our coffees on the wall, we're able to climb over a low railing, stepping carefully through shrubbery to find ourselves face-to-face with a statue of a woman whose raised arm is part greeting, part warning. The lawn is bordered with tulips that are a dusty deep purple, almost black. There are benches, too, the very proper kind with dividers between each seat. Side by side, divided, we sip our coffee. The night sky is clear, framed by new-leafed trees.

We laugh and talk and laugh some more. I learn (and promptly forget) the Spanish word for *caterpillar*. I learn that there are possums in Los Angeles. I learn that the Quiet Guy loves being an uncle. We talk about turning thirty, which he said for him was about becoming sensible. "That clearly doesn't apply abroad," he adds, smiling.

After a while, the benches grow so uncomfortable that we move to the lawn, lying spread out as if it were a summer's afternoon. Gulls wheel ghostly pale against the sky, which is a luminous midnight blue though it must be around five A.M.

"Won't you lay your head here?" he asks, as I try to make the clutch that I've been using as a cushion into a kindlier shape. I lie back down, and gently he maneuvers us so that his chest is pillowing me. The warmth makes us realize how cold we've become, but our shivers are partly tiredness, partly the delight of contact after hours and hours of tantalizing proximity. It's not the same as the fit between Jake and me, but we two fit in another way—we fit conversationally. We stay like that awhile, newly bashful, and part of me wishes that nothing more will happen. Wouldn't that make it most special of all?

But there is something more to my desire to go no further, something besides chaste good behavior. Over Christmas, the Quiet Guy had sent me an e-mail describing his holidays and mentioning—in passing and without further explanation—some "future in-laws." He's engaged! I thought. It explained quite a bit. But no sooner had I thought it than I began thinking of other possible explanations. Maybe they were a sibling's future in-laws and it was just a big, inclusive Southern thing, referring to them as your own. It sounded desperate even to me, but I couldn't imagine why, if he was engaged, he hadn't brought it up before, more explicitly.

I'm on the verge of asking him about it when he takes my hand. "We should have done this ages ago," he says, and I try to joke about it, replying that it feels so lovely, we might drift off like this. Wouldn't it be alarming to wake in a park together? "We'd find a way to laugh about it," he says, and I have to admit he's right. We don't fall asleep but we do fall quiet, lightly holding each other as dawn arrives on a cool breeze and red-eyes score a grid of vapor trails across the whitening sky.

To question him would be to shatter the spell, and I can't quite bring myself to think that such a kind, funny, decent man would behave like this if he really were promised to another. Had I learned nothing from all those twentysomething mishaps? Not much, it would seem. Even so, a part of me breathes a sigh of relief. Misguided I may be, but at least I retain a bit of optimism, even if it's less innocent than downright naïve.

A nearby clock strikes seven, and only then do we kiss—it is tender, thoughtful. Eventually, a dog walker in a quilted jacket bustles in. He looks amused to see us, and the Quiet Guy quickly tidies away our cups in an effort to make our scene look a little more respectable. "Crazy people love coffee," he says, smiling. He doesn't know the half of it.

ELEVEN

April in New York OR *Chasing Tales*

An unattempted woman cannot boast of her chastity.
—Michel de Montaigne

When I run, New York is the place I run to, and this time is no
different. I'm here for a week, and though I've arranged a
sublet in Hell's Kitchen, it won't be ready until tomorrow, so tonight
will be spent in the Beau's pied-à-terre, a loft with just one bed. It's a
very big bed, he promises, and I've decided to take him at his word.
Besides, after all those nocturnal tussles with Jake, the $250 cost of a
hotel room seems a pretty steep price to place on my tattered chastity.

I ended up going to the airport directly from another early-hours
radio stint. As I wheeled a large red suitcase into the studio, it struck
me that this was precisely the kind of scenario I'd have craved a few
years ago: on air, in air, too busy for sleep. The glamour was already
wearing thin after a few predawn hours at Heathrow, and by the
time the suitcase and I trundle through immigration, I feel like I've
been up for weeks.

New York is hot—unseasonably, sweatily so. The Beau has bid me meet him downtown, in the lobby of a trendily made-over hotel. He isn't due for another hour, so I decide to freshen up and grab some lunch. After a humiliating few minutes spent trying to extract a change of clothes from my suitcase and instead pulling out everything else, right there in the middle of the lobby, I leave my luggage in the cloakroom and make for the bathroom. My reflection in the mirror is haggard, and for a panicky few minutes I'm trapped by the room's minimalist design, which disguises doors as walls.

The restaurant is full of people winding up lunch meetings, looking to close deals as they knock back espressos and wave for the bill. There are no windows here and each table is an island, illuminated by its own spotlight. It's a bit like being on a stage, except that we're all too busy watching ourselves to be one another's audience. Music discreetly covers the hum of conversation—a mournful Middle Eastern voice, swooping around an excitable drumbeat. I order a salad, and a complicated arrangement of leaves and spears arrives— a gastronomic pick-up sticks. It's all too much on so little sleep. Looking for escape, I open the novel I've brought with me.

It starts with a girl sitting alone at a restaurant table. Ha! I think. Fancy that. And I take a sip of water. In the next sentence, the girl in the story does exactly that. It's the first page of the novel, but already she's caught up in some kind of existential crisis. Overcaffeinated and underslept, I'm seized by the vertiginous sense that this life is not quite mine. Just as I'm feeling thoroughly spooked, I feel a hand on my shoulder and jump. It is the Beau, dapper and smiling, ready to sweep me downtown.

Can sweeping be done by subway? Not with a suitcase this huge. This may not be the life I'm meant to be leading, but while I'm here,

I may as well do things in style. He insists on a cab, and we stutter through the Midtown traffic.

During the four and a half hours that I spent at the deserted airport, a series of e-mails popped up on my BlackBerry to keep me awake. Some were from the Beau, wanting to know which flight I was on and checking that I had his phone number—touching but disconcertingly parental. Others were from Quiet Guy, who happened also to be bound for New York on business. To one message, he attached a photo taken with his phone: a rainbow arcing through a gray sky, landing on a sign that read GOLDEN ANGEL PANCAKE HOUSE, OPEN 24 HOURS. On the other side of the Atlantic, we missed each other by two hours at Kennedy Airport. As he was heading into the city, he warned me that he was feeling as though he had slept in a park.

We're to meet in a café just as soon as I've checked into the Hotel du Beau, but it's so nice out, we grab iced teas and stroll toward Central Park instead. The season has lurched overnight from late winter to late spring, bringing out everyone and everything. How strange to see tulips blooming in such heat, and not the dark tulips of our London park but big, blowsy American tulips. We chat aimlessly until the Quiet Guy looks away, fixing his eyes on the ground. "So, there's something I have to tell you," he says, and with these few, heart-plunging words he conveys pretty much all I need to know.

"I know," I say, and truly I do—now and probably from the start. Isn't it always the quiet ones whom you're meant to watch? That slight reticence I'd sensed and tried to attribute to shyness—or even, desperately, gayness—it obviously meant just one thing.

He is engaged.

While he stumbles through the beginnings of an apology and then veers off toward self-justification, I glance sideways at him and see those neat features of his twitching to compose a face that might befit this situation—no doubt new and strange to him, but wearisomely familiar to me.

He gardens and wears squishy suede shoes and applies lip balm in a frankly girlie way. And did I mention that he's engaged? (Did *he* mention that he's engaged?) For all these reasons and more, we do not belong together. Oh, but then there is the way he lets those languid Southern vowels detain his speech. Hearing him say a humdrum word like *pine,* for instance—it's aural hypnotism. But he is engaged. One of the many ironies is that it was the vow that led me to him. I'd congratulated myself on tuning in to a subtler serenade, when in reality it was subtle for the very good reason that he is unavailable. Being virtuous of intent does not necessarily lead to virtuous deeds, it seems.

Just then, a gust of blossom sweeps across our little scene. Settling on our shoulders like pink confetti, it's joyously mocking as we lean against the railings, sulkily slurping our iced teas amid the street performers and hustlers. Afterward, we stroll back to his company's office together. He's promised to print off some material that I need for work, but I'm sure he's thinking as I am: that it might help reposition our friendship on safer ground. As we cross a street, something funny happens—something very New York: four young, shirtless male joggers appear, making straight for us—or for me, as the Quiet Guy points out. Trampled by bare-chested boys—what a way to go! We're still laughing about it as we step into his office.

·   ·   ·

Later, sitting with more iced tea in a cool, empty bar, I reflect that I've been in the city barely five hours and have already managed to whip up an emotional storm. I am a liability. In the background is the mix tape of all mix tapes: Dylan, Lennon, Dolly Parton—their voices fill the air with jealousy and longing and regret. Beyond, children and paunchy old men and middle-aged ladies in linen stroll by—a panorama of the blameless, though it would be wrong to believe that their lives were untouched by such churning sentiments, just as I was wrong to expect that knocking sex from the equation would in any way exempt me. And what of the Quiet Guy's fiancée? How would it feel to find out that your intended had spent a lost night in a foreign city with another woman? Would it matter that there was no sex when instead there was laughter, talk, shared quietness—not to mention rainbows sent soaring across the Atlantic?

That evening, I stroll out to dinner with the Beau. He's wearing a stripy sports jacket and I'm in a candy-barred blouse. Our accidental coordination coaxes a smile to my face, and he listens as I tell him all about the fiasco with the Quiet Guy. Though the sun has dropped in the sky, its warmth lingers on the sidewalks and in the atmosphere—summery diners spill out of restaurants whose fronts have opened up to the street, even though it isn't yet May. The sense that this might all be a passing mirage—that it still could snow next week—seems to have given everyone holiday license.

Afterward, for the third time in the space of a week, I find myself lying horizontal with a man—a third man. The first was on a sofa with Jake, a messy tangle of limbs and clothes, breathless and regrettable.

The second was al fresco. And now there's an actual bed involved. Sweeping aside for a moment the profound unsuitability of each, I wonder whether chastity mightn't be a novel dating strategy. There's also the worry that some puckish god of romance has decided to play a joke on me, dispatching several years' worth of suitors all at once, knowing that I'm unable to make the most of even the single ones. Perhaps this current dry spell will merely prove the warm-up to an epic involuntary drought? But while I should feel spoiled, I'm mostly confused. If this were a novel, it wouldn't hang together at all well. There's just too much going on for any coherent plot to emerge. It is meant to be my story, yet the men are running away with it.

The bed is, as promised, enormous—possibly the hugest I've ever seen. Two people could very easily lose each other on its espresso-sheeted expanse. A third could be snuck in and nobody need know. Had those fabled ten, little one and all, snuggled up here for the night, there would never have been a nursery rhyme. But while the bed's dimensions are assuredly chaste, they also make it much harder to ignore. This isn't just a bed, it's a B-E-D.

"Is this weird?" asks the Beau, stretching his hand out across the empty swath that separates us. If I stretched out mine, would it reach his? We go to bed with other people wanting so many different things. It's rare that we get them, but tonight, I feel like I'm getting exactly what I want: to close my eyes in the company of a dear friend who knows my best sides and my worst—a platonic friend in the truest sense of the word.

Later, I receive a predawn wake-up call in the form of smashing glass as a precariously balanced vase meets its end in the bathroom sink. I listen for a few minutes to the sound of someone trying to be quiet, followed by the noise of the apartment door closing softly. It is four A.M.

Over a diner breakfast a reasonable number of hours later, the Beau tells me that he'd taken himself off to an all-night café. He often wakes at dawn, I know, but I find that I'm glad we weren't able to last a whole night together, sleeping chastely side by side. I may have his insomnia to thank for it, but the Beau's flight from the humongous bed preserved a possibility that I now sense anchors our friendship. While he leans companionably over to finish the bacon I've left, I return to my tea and tabloid.

My sublet is so tiny, there is barely room to open my suitcase. There is barely room for me. Every surface, every nook and cranny, is festooned with stuff. It's such a weird and wild assortment of belongings that it's impossible to be any more precise, though I detect a vaguely Edwardian theme to the clutter. The entire apartment could be tucked up in the Beau's bed with room to spare. Its owner is off at a meditation retreat where there are no computers, no mobile phones and no words. It is a totally silent retreat, and she is hoping it will cure her writer's block. On a table, she has left me one of her published short stories, a modest stack of photocopied pages with a pleasant note attached. Stepping round it, I switch on the TV to catch the news. A Hollywood actor has kissed a Bollywood actress at a televised awards ceremony in India and caused a national uproar. It's a reminder that kisses are not to be taken for granted.

After my freakishly glorious arrival afternoon, it rains and rains. I walk everywhere and get drenched. Right now, I'm walking very quickly, still getting drenched, and can feel blisters blooming on my heels. Along with an umbrella, I'm clutching three hairy-stalked sunflowers, heads lolling in dismay at the deluge, and a soggy scrap of paper bearing an obscure private address on the far Upper West Side. As I near the river, the city begins to trail off, its rigid grid yielding to curves and dead ends.

As luck would have it, the Pasha is also in town and has invited me to a dinner party. The only other guest when I arrive is a sometime girlfriend of his, a vivacious postgrad anthropologist still firmly in her twenties.

"I've heard so much about you," she says, youth's radiant confidence flooding her smile as she shakes my hand. What do I really think of those age gaps? It's hard for me to disapprove after my dalliance with the Beau, and I've been lectured often enough about how in my own case it stems from a nonexistent relationship with my father. There's probably some truth to that, but then again, I know plenty of women who are the products of perfectly functional father-daughter relationships and yet still find themselves entangled with older men. My theory is this—and it's one that I whisper because it sounds so retrograde: we still yearn to defer to the men we're involved with. Up until the middle of the last century, we'd have done so simply because they were men, because they controlled our finances and because their destinies were ours. We're not going to do that again, but age and experience and achievement remain permissible.

The Pasha's dinner is fun. More people turn up than there are seats, but there is a plateful of risotto for everyone and plenty of good red wine. I end up staying late, chatting to a friend of the vivacious anthropologist. A big girl with bold features and enough aplomb to carry it all off, she tells me a story that makes me feel older but not necessarily wiser, that makes me a little wistful but also makes me smile. She has an ex passing through town, she says. He's going to be in New York for only one night and, in a surreal twist, is flush with cash he has won on a TV quiz show. She can't decide whether to hook up with him or not, though even as she tells me this, she checks her watch, suggesting that she knows exactly what she'll do.

Would I have done the same at her age? Like her, I'd have undoubtedly gone through all the motions of pretending that I might not make that booty call, that I might not sleep with a guy I'd ruled out any future with. Despite her buxom sass, this bright young woman still feels the need to be coy about her desires—it's part of the fun, though I can imagine running into her tomorrow evening and hearing a very different take on it all. It occurs to me that we seduce ourselves with the potency of our own sexuality—seduce ourselves away from other truths and desires.

I see the Pasha once more before I leave New York. He accompanies me to dinner with some work friends of mine in Cobble Hill, and we cab back across the river together, remembering that one of Brooklyn's great pluses is that you get to return to the island afterward, cruising across the bridge and back into Manhattan's gleaming embrace. Smitten anew by all that twinkly beauty, we decide to stop for one final drink in a tiny tavern—the kind of place you know you'll never be able to find in daylight hours. Perched on stools, we sip bourbon, savoring the cool clunk of ice cubes, the slight caramel tang. The music is loud and the bar's sticky surface tells a thousand and one tales.

Just as I'm beginning to think how nice it is, after all the dramas that we two have shared—breaking up on my birthday, for instance—to be able to prop up the bar like this, we wend our way round to the subject of that same breakup. It probably shouldn't be surprising that we turn out to tell the story so differently, but the vehemence with which we defend our versions takes me aback.

"You pursued me!" That's him, astonishingly.

"You pursued *me*!" That's me—rhetoric has never been a strong suit.

"Well, I was in no position to—"

"And how was I meant to have known that?" I interrupt—a bad habit, granted, but in this instance I feel justified.

"Intuition."

Intuition? Now I'm furious. "You got what you wanted and got it guilt-free—because I was meant to have used my *intuition*?" I'm not sure how we got here, and I know that I've backed myself into a line of argument that I don't entirely endorse, but it's late—very, very late—and alcohol has been consumed. What I'm telling him, I realize, is that he got to sleep with me—implying that that wasn't what I, too, wanted. It was, though I wanted other things as well. I wanted commitment, I wanted security, I wanted devotion. If my line of argument conjures up prefeminist specters of female sexuality—of its nonexistence, essentially—then his draws on something far more ancient: the myth of the feminine sixth sense.

In the end, I'm saved by the Pasha's more recent ex. Having not eaten, she has been out drinking and is now in a cab with no money. The bar is cell-phone free, and as the Pasha's drama unfolds, garbled, teary call after call, he has to keep darting in and out, where it is once again pouring. Perhaps their relationship isn't quite the ancient history that I'd assumed it to be. Or perhaps she's decided, like me, that tonight is the night for comparing notes on their breakup. Ducking back in, the Pasha announces that he has to go find her, leaving me to pick up the tab and hail a cab. As I sail uptown in my yellow tub, I glimpse the two of them—she huddled in a doorway, he pacing the pavement, hands thrust deep in his pockets. They're not looking bewitched but seem amply bothered and bewildered. Bedraggled, too. Sinking back in my seat, I thank Cupid that this is one drama in which I'm not starring. What a relief to be an onlooker for once, free to leave whenever I wish.

The driver has the radio tuned to an early-hours phone-in show, and as we swish through the sodden city, I listen to a woman caller complain that after a year, her man still doesn't want kids. The host cuts in to tell her how it is. But how is it, really? Here is what I know this wet Manhattan evening: that once you've had sex with a man, it's hard not to fall for the fairy-tale extras. That it is such a powerful thing, its spell lingers long, long after you last embraced, tugging your heart—and, given enough liquor lubrication, your tongue, too—back to those torrid intimacies in all their heated irrationality.

Back at my Hell's Kitchen sublet, I finally pick up the story that my landlady's left out for me to read. It is a romance.

TWELVE

May and June OR *Vive la Différence!*

> The most virtuous women have something
> within them, something that is never chaste.
>
> —Honoré de Balzac, *The Physiology of Marriage*

Eight months ago, if I'd had the nerve to squint ahead from the start line and imagine—really imagine—what this long year might be like, I'd have guessed that the hardest stretch would have been around about now. So close to the finish line and yet weeks away—weeks and weeks and weeks. Instead, it feels like I'm just beginning.

Of course, I didn't really know what I was giving up when I decided upon my vow. Sex means different things to different people at different times: it cannot signify the same hopes or satisfy the same yearnings for the eighteen-year-old as it does for the twenty-eight- or the fifty-eight- or the eighty-eight-year-old.

Removing sex from my own life has left a bigger, differently shaped hole than I would have imagined. The physical withdrawal is acute at times, but it passes. What is it that the abstinence primers suggest? Go for a jog? It mostly works. I can see that sex was a dis-traction that allowed me to ignore pretty much everything else in my life that wasn't quite what it should or could have been. I became fixated on relationships to the exclusion of friendships, family or any sense of where I was headed. It wasn't so much about the sex itself, but it was the sex that gave those affairs badly needed sub-stance. Without it, their stories weren't fully absorbing. Over these past few weeks, I've skittered along their surfaces like—well, like an addict looking for a fix, longing to be engulfed by the old, familiar drama.

If only we could do without sex. *New Yorker* writers James Thurber and E. B. White agreed in their best-selling book, *Is Sex Necessary?* A spoof classic from 1929 (its publication coincided with the Wall Street crash), it was inspired by the burgeoning sales of pseudosci-entific tomes. "Doctors, psychiatrists and other students of misbe-havior were pursuing sex to the last ditch and the human animal seemed absorbed in self-analysis," White noted in an introduction. In the decades since, pop culture has apparently managed to strip love from sex, but we still don't really believe in love *without* sex. In marriage, nonconsummation remains grounds for annulment in certain situations. Friendship hasn't escaped sexualization, either. Platonic? "The sex part always gets in the way," Billy Crystal's char-acter insists in *When Harry Met Sally*. And when it doesn't get in the way, that untapped potential—that sexual frisson—seems somehow necessary, however one-sided. Take the Beau and me. I like that we're platonic but hate the thought that we might have settled the matter once and for all. Ours is a kind of courtly love, I sometimes joke, though in fact academics are still squabbling over whether even that was as chaste as legend has it. Chaste or not, its ballads still rely on an erotic charge.

Sex has been disguising something, and it's only in the middle of the night, midway across the Atlantic, that I'm finally forced to acknowledge it. Despite making the final base off limits, I've nevertheless spent two-thirds of my chaste year in pursuit of the emotional turbulence that went with it. Perhaps it's not my relationship with sex that is the problem, but my relationship with male attention. Exhausted and overwrought, buzzing with too much sugar and caffeine, and softened up by the tearjerker movie that I watched while the other passengers slept, I find myself sobbing silently into my red fleece American Airlines blanket.

This is the moment a shrink would ask me about my father. And what about him? Though he lived with my mother and sister and me until I was sixteen, he wasn't part of our life. When we moved to the house where I spent most of my childhood, the first thing I remember him doing was fitting a lock on the door of the room that was to be his studio. He kept different hours from us, and whenever he was cajoled into taking part in family life—a school play, for instance—he would find something to do beforehand that would guarantee he'd arrive late. There are a few better memories, but their scarcity makes them sharp and strange.

On the plus side, his presence, however absent, ensured that there was no scope for my sister or me to build up an idealized portrait of the father we might have had. He was right there—or in his studio, at any rate—to refute it. At primary school, I learned that other people's fathers weren't the same. I remember drawing up a bossy curriculum of "Dad lessons," and then, when he failed to show any improvement, miming a lobotomy. That also failed, so I turned around and got on with my six-year-old's life.

Could I blame him for the fact that I've failed to sustain a significant romance since college? Possibly, but it would be a cop-out.

After all, my sister has conducted her affairs very differently. In truth, our mother parented for two, and we didn't feel we were missing anything. What I will say is that not having had a real father has probably left me ill-equipped to deal with male attention.

A short while ago, I interviewed Germaine Greer and she mentioned that Italian women know exactly how to deal with it. They accept it as their due; they don't feel obliged to take it anywhere. For us British women, it's a far less frequent occurrence, and if we don't grow up with it, it can be disconcertingly intoxicating. I can trace the first time I really became aware of it to a precise instant, though the details surrounding it have faded out of remembrance.

It was on a residential school trip to a nearby country estate so long used for such things that the smell of school dinners and teenage sweat had become ingrained, masking any trace of former glory. We were there for two or three days of wholesome outdoorsy activities like orienteering and obstacle courses. There must have been a curfew in the evening, but for a few hours after dinner we were left to hang out with the vending machines and dartboards.

There I was, standing with another girl watching two boys play Ping-Pong. I've forgotten their faces and names; I just remember laughing a little too hard at something one of them said—my nerves rather than their wit. Suddenly the boys' eyes were on me, but in addition to the usual mortification—I was a girl whose whole school career was spent trying to blend—I felt a ripple of something very like power. They weren't mocking me, I saw. Instead, it was as if they'd noticed me for the first time. Earlier that day, I'd surprised myself by taking the lead in our orienteering team, and though my cheeks flushed as the Ping-Pong ball resumed its to-ing and fro-ing across the net, I glowed with a feeling that in some small, essential way resembled the feeling of possessing compass if not map.

All of this drifts to mind as the plane cruises through timeless darkness back toward a London dawn, casting my headlong pursuit of male attention in an uncomfortable light.

Would I have slept with any of these men if I could have? I suspect that, yes, I probably would have slept with one of them, and in the dizzy drama that followed, I wouldn't have spotted this greediness in myself. There is something insatiable about my appetite for male indulgence. I get giddy on it, losing sight of whatever it was I might have wanted, and losing, too, my ability to judge the genuine from the tactical on their part. To really give chastity a go, I need to wean myself off a certain kind of male attention. By the time the air hostesses bring breakfast round, I'm bug-eyed with tiredness and tears, but I've also renewed my vow.

When we land, there it is waiting for me, my first test: Jake, as timely as ever. Well, not Jake himself, but a date to a film screening with him. Should I cancel? Probably, but, delirious with fatigue and the exhilaration of midair revelations, I decide I can deal with the challenge. The invitation had arrived while I was in New York, and is a first from him. Yes, I'd replied, due back that morning. Tapping out the email, my fingernails a freshly painted neon pink that I'd never have worn in London, I'd momentarily believed myself the kind of girl who'd sashay into the cinema lobby, kiss him on the cheek and just be cool with how things are between us.

I will never be that girl, not with Jake, though I do better than you might imagine. The jet lag probably helps, casting a dreamy veil over everything—even the movie, which turns out to be a horror film based on a translation by a friend of Jake's. Too tired to drop my gaze or even blink, I watch all the gory bits. I even see the moment where the film's male lead (hero he isn't) hides behind a locked door, listening to his wife pounding on the other side, screaming to be let in as virus-infected baddies eat her alive. Who'd want a husband like that? I think. And then: Could Jake do that? I glance over at him and his expression isn't reassuring.

The evening has grown chilly by the time we leave, ducking down a side alley and into a Soho club. Jake is fielding calls from abroad and keeps diving out to answer his phone. In between we chat, and I find myself telling him something that I haven't yet told you: I've decided to return to New York for three whole months.

It's something I've talked and talked about over the years. After all, who wouldn't want to live in New York? Actually, I, for one. My initial infatuation ebbed a while back, but in its place has grown a fondness for the city's less noticeable traits—not its speed but its solidity. People walk at my pace—quick, very quick—yet certain things endure. The *New York Times* masthead, for instance. Galoshes. Ma'am. The city may clunk and steam and hiss alarmingly, the pavements may be in such a lousy state of disrepair that you expect them to sprout saplings at any moment, but mostly it works, and it works especially well—perhaps too well—if you are a single woman. All the consolations you could want are right there.

I still remember my first trip to the city, alone and knowing almost nobody. I walked everywhere. I ate pizza slices and knishes, and on open-late evening at the Met sat sipping an apple martini, unself-consciously on my own. I looked and I listened and I was there on the magical first day of summer, when the temperature leaped up and suddenly the umbrella sellers were hawking ice water. There were flashes of loneliness, but they weren't merely bearable, they were poetic. Despite the crowded torridity of the past week, I continue to think of New York as a place of solitude both healing and inspiring.

Being briefly absent from London has made me realize that I've changed these past months—outgrown the small city that I've made of it, a pocket-handkerchief metropolis hemmed in by favorite parks and tea shops. In order to redraw it, I need more time away, and where better to go than New York? As E. B. White put it in his classic essay "Here is New York," "You always feel that either by shifting your location ten blocks or by reducing your fortune by five dollars you can experience rejuvenation." Wasn't that what I was doing when I counted out exactly five dollars for my sparkly ring? New York is the city that I love above all others, and if chastity cannot take me to a man I'll love and be loved back by, perhaps it can lead to a place instead—the very place where this quest began.

For all these reasons, the idea of relocation had sidled up to me anew: I could pack up my books in London, hand in notice to my landlady, and return for a longer spell. There is one more reason why the plan appeals, and he's lounging across from me—Jake.

So though I omit that last bit, I'm not fibbing when I tell him of my plans, and while it would be gratifying to see a flash of something—surprise, if not regret—I find that I don't want him to dissuade me. Telling him, I realize that I truly have made up my mind. He walks me to the bus stop afterward, and when my bus arrives, I step aboard and don't look back.

There is a long and outlandish tradition of men renouncing sex in order to conserve semen, which has in turn been the focus of obsessive study by everyone from philosophers to sports coaches. Historically, intercourse has been far more imperiling for women—for centuries, pregnancy took as well as gave life, while the stigma of ruination could lead to destitution and other grim fates—yet it is men who have traditionally been warned off it for medical reasons.

Hippocrates, for instance, taught that women required semen in order to keep their wombs happy. "Hysterical" symptoms were caused by an upset womb crying out for sex. At the same time, he advised men to preserve their stores of semen, which was deemed essential to male vitality.

In Hinduism, a strand of thought links semen's preservation to health as well as to spiritual and moral development. As Elizabeth Abbott notes in *A History of Celibacy,* "In no other religion is the power of semen as pronounced as in Hinduism and related religious traditions. Semen is a vital fluid, the essence of life." She goes on to explain that in one set of Hindu sacred texts, the Upanishads, its loss is mourned as a kind of death. To produce a single drop requires the essence of sixty drops of blood. (According to these same texts, intercourse not only weakens but shortens human lives, because the number of breaths each person will take over the course of a lifetime is fixed at birth, and all that rapid panting hastens things along.)

Victorian thriftiness allied sexual continence to profitable industriousness, and professional athletes bound for Grecian arenas and modern-day soccer fields alike have advocated sex bans.

But what is the payoff when a woman abstains? Female sexuality is riddling. Anatomically, our signs of arousal and climax are sphinx-like compared with the upfront razzmatazz of erection and ejaculation. As Freud famously confessed to a female student, "The great question that has never been answered and which I have not yet been able to answer, despite my 30 years of research into the feminine soul, is, What does a woman want?" Almost a century later, the search continues, generating flurries of research papers and filling the pages of esteemed journals, both psychoanalytical and scientific.

When we swear off sex, do we also reap rewards of increased potency, and how would that manifest itself? If centuries of codified fear of female sexuality are anything to go by, it must be something mighty and awe-inspiring.

It's a small thing, but I'm certain that without my vow, I would never have made this much-mooted decision to relocate across the Atlantic. "This decisiveness—it's all very uncharacteristic," a colleague points out over lunch, peering at me suspiciously. "You haven't been reading self-help books, have you?"

After talking about making such a move for years, it seems strange that it is actually happening. I know that the decision was mine, but already it has acquired autonomy. I've handed in notice to my landlady and cleared it with my editors. I'm looking for storage here and a sublet there. It's only for a few months, but things are dismantling around me—at first intangibles like the sense of stability; later, shelves, cupboards, towers of books that have sat on the coffee table long enough to make their mark, a deeper-hued patch on a sun-bleached surface.

It's this same decisiveness that prompts me to say yes when, a few weeks later, my screenwriter friend Dave invites me to Cannes, where he's been working on some rewrites. My male friendships are numerous, and until now it hasn't occurred to me to question them. But this particular one is trouble-free, and if it counts as male attention, it's of a far less problematic kind. Dave's wife, Nat, is glamorous, funny and nifty with a sword (she fences in her spare time). She's also a high-powered banker in the middle of closing a hairy deal, and he is desperate for some English-language chat.

I spend a couple of days sitting on the sunny balcony of their apartment, reading and writing and thinking about the chaos that I've created back in London. In the evenings, we drink sensational supermarket reds and eat deep-fried zucchini flowers. Dave's screenplays are full of sex, and at one restaurant, sitting at a pavement table, we begin arguing loudly about it all. We're having fun—somehow, just being in France lends the subject a gravitas that it wouldn't have had back home, even if what we were saying had been ten times smarter.

"What about Simone de Beauvoir?" I demand. "She was all talk. I mean, she spent most of her time weeping over Sartre, and if not him, then some other man." Dave laughs. However seriously our host nation takes it, we're not taking it very seriously at all. Still, over the past months, this is something that has been nagging at me. Not the French (though I am fascinated by how Frenchwomen keep their sexy myth going), nor Simone de Beauvoir (though it's true that she did do a lot of weeping in cafés), but the problem of feminism.

Much of what my chaste experience has shown me seems to fly directly in the face of feminist teachings—or at least feminist teachings as we think of them. The idea that it's more empowering to be the pursued rather than the pursuer, for instance. Or that as women, sex is something to use as a bartering chip, withholding it to win compliments, courtship, commitment. So many of these lessons rest on the notion that there are differences—fundamental differences— in the way men and women experience sex, and that notion itself seems to have become taboo.

From a certain perspective, gender equality doesn't look much like equality at all. We've earned the right to work and play like men, but even those victories, questioned by many a working mum, are local—we haven't made the world a significantly easier place for our sisters in Africa or the Middle East; we haven't made the world any more female. Do we even know what that means? While a gussied-up parody of femininity is everywhere, we've lost sight of femaleness.

A while ago, I spent some time living in Paris. I was curious about the erotic power of the Frenchwoman—how does she keep such a potent cultural stereotype alive? A thirtysomething French lawyer with London dating experience seemed like he might be able to provide clues. With an Englishwoman, he told me, there is no need to try imagining what it might be like to sleep with her. Her charms are all there on the surface, and they're not terribly alluring at that. "Who wants to go to bed with a drunk mermaid?" he said with a smile, proving that the Gallic male is all about seduction even when he's being insulting.

It's seduction that we Englishwomen fail at, my companion explained. The French pride themselves on it, while across the Channel we simply raise a glass or ten and hope for the best. Seduction is a striptease that's both physical and psychological, and its charge rests in the hidden—it's all about keeping something back, holding out for as long as possible before revealing the full monty. Even the most obviously self-parodying kinky underwear hides a little something— a nipple, say. Adam's and Eve's demure fig leaves are precisely what make you think of that juicy apple. Total nudity, as anyone who's ever strayed onto a nudist beach knows, is rarely erotic.

The other thing that the French aren't shy about is gender distinctions. Does it help that it's ingrained in their grammar? In English, our nouns are sexless, but gender roles are still encoded in our romantic vocabulary, and it makes us wary.

It's actually what Tracy and Hepburn were trying to figure out all those years ago as feuding husband-and-wife lawyers in *Adam's Rib*.

"Vive la différence!" cheers Tracy's Adam, reunited with Hepburn's Amanda at the film's end. "Which means?" she asks—though there's always a sense that she knows, of course she knows, she's just testing him. "Which means hurrah for that little difference," he answers.

Meanwhile, the messy business of feelings and desire has acted as a constant and inconvenient reminder to feminists that a difference does indeed exist. It keeps ambushing them and contradicting their finely reasoned treatises. Even Simone fell in love over and over. Feminist Lynne Segal writes of how her own fantasies of being overwhelmed by a man jangled uneasily with the doctrines she was passionate about, and wryly relates the tale of another woman so turned on by images shown at an antipornography screening that she actually became gay. "Desire still refused to obey principled rules; least of all, our rules," Segal notes.

From Nice, I'm brought back to reality with a cold, wet thud when I'm sent west to cover a music festival. After that weird flash of New York summer and the Côte d'Azur sunshine, Britain feels chilly, but spring has finally sprung. Perhaps its lateness accounts for its lushness, because even London is swathed in green. Buds burst open, dogs give chase on the common, and pigeons flirt, puffing themselves up and hopping bashfully along the rooftop opposite my desk. Heading out of the city, the view is even greener. As it scrolls beyond the train window, it spells a single word: fertile.

N, the musician, has invited me to stay the weekend at his uncle's house in the Quantock Hills, close to the festival. After camping at this same festival the year before, I leap at the chance, and it's not until somewhere beyond Swindon that the situation's potential awkwardness registers. This might be seen as a kind of first date—

a residential first date, with assorted musical grandees as onlookers. It could be awful. As the train pushes onward, a fine mist begins to fall—the gentle, unhurried rain that tells you it's going nowhere anytime soon.

At Bath, I change trains and head deeper into the West Country. N is to meet me at the nearest station. I'd expected him to be late, but when I step onto the platform, I spot him leaning against a mud-spattered car. He is wearing a plaid shirt and dark shades—part young farmer, part rock star—and waving uncertainly, as if one or the other of us might be a mirage. "You're in my hands now," he tells me, holding them out and shrugging slightly as I wander over.

The station turns out to have been nearby only in the rural sense. Some forty minutes later, we pull into a graveled driveway and wind our way up to a proud-looking Georgian rectory. N has clearly had the same thought as I—this could be awful—and has taken the precaution of inviting along another friend, a banjo player, no less, who is expected anytime now. We three will be staying in the converted stables next door, N explains. A sleepover, I think, and realize that it won't be terrible.

Lunch is pleasantly chaotic, enlivened by a pack of aging spaniels, still sprightly enough to make them hard to number. While we wait for the Banjo Player to turn up, N takes me on a tour of the surrounding hamlet. In borrowed wellies, I clamber over a stile and follow him down to the bottom of a sodden pasture where a stream rushes. Over the years, I've buried my rural roots so effectively that most people assume I grew up in London. In wellies, there's no disguising the country in me, and N shoots me a surprised look, reappraising the little he knows.

As we lean over a bridge, a pair of small birds flit close by. Conversation hasn't been a problem, but alone by the gurgling stream and the chirruping birds—lovebirds, for heaven's sake!—it dries up. "Let's play Poohsticks," N says. We each drop our twig into the water and they vanish beneath the bridge. When they emerge, neither is winning. Churned up in the current, they have become locked together. Together, they sail away. Birds do it, bees do it, even twigs do it. The hills are so steep that wherever I look, greenness fills my vision, dotted with frolicking white lambs. You could get drunk on all this verdure. It's as if the natural world is screaming at us to kick off our wellies, tear off our big woolly pullovers, and get down to fornicating right there on the muddy banks of the stream. Just then, a shout comes from up on the lane: saved by the Banjo Player.

Later that night there is a big party at the house. A couple of decades shy of the average age—locals outnumber festival-goers—we three feel like kids again. We've dressed up, N in a suit of saffron moleskin and me in my red heels that keep sinking into the turf. The Banjo Player has dug out a Nehru shirt, which, coupled with his closely cropped hair, gives him the look of a New Age guru. While he talks ukuleles with a raven-haired hippie, N beckons me into the kitchen, where some ladies from the village are doling out steaming lamb stew. Grabbing a couple of plates and topping up our tumblers of red wine, he leads the way out into the dusk.

The damp, chilly dusk.

We dine at a picnic table, with umbrellas instead of a parasol. The romance of N's plan, helped a bit by the moleskin jacket that is now draped over my shoulders, means I barely shiver at all. New arrivals pick their way down the path and sheep call from the hills. With rain pattering overhead, we clink glasses. As first dates go, it isn't bad.

Back at the stables, it seems that my room, with its cozy quilt, wall of paperbacks and woody scent, is usually N's. While the Banjo

Player is sleeping down the hallway, selfless N is bedding down in a nook between the door and the boiler. I go to sleep feeling a tiny bit guilty about all the empty space in my bed.

It rains pretty much the whole weekend, but on Saturday it pours. The festival site is awash with mud and I splash around in my wellies. That evening, we regroup for leftover lamb stew. Far from feeling awkward, the situation is growing more and more comfortable. Seeing a person in the context of his friends is incredibly informative. N and I haven't even kissed, but he's made me tea and toast, offered to carry me over puddles and mocked my aversion to rural life. Already I feel closer to him than to plenty of the men I've slept with. But could I see myself with him? The answer remains no, though the question presents itself with increasing frequency.

After supper we head off into the sodden countryside, bound for a surreally fancy party complete with champagne, seafood and burlesque, none of which quite obscures the fact that we're in a big tent in a field. N and I circle each other for most of the evening, and when the music starts, he hits the dance floor with some eccentric moves that neither I nor my colleague Caitlin, whom I find skulking by the lobster, can interpret. Is he beckoning us to join or shooing us away?

"He your boyfriend, then?" she asks, nodding toward him in an appraising—and, yes, slyly admiring—kind of way. "Oh, no," I say, ashamed by the haste of my reply. "He's just . . . a friend. I'm staying with him," I explain. But later on, when I spot him flirting with a woman in leather trousers, I wander over and stand next to him as if I were.

Sitting beside me on the way back to the rectory, he brushes something from the hem of my skirt, his fingers skimming my knee, lingering momentarily. I don't move, but nor do I flinch. And then they're gone. I look over and, in the dark, smile into his eyes—a smile of gratitude for all his gestures of offbeat romance bestowed without the expectation of anything in return. Then again, if it's a canny ploy, it may just be working. Like a crazy idea, I can see how he might grow on a person.

It's almost dawn by the time we roll up at the stables, where N pours three nightcaps. The rain has briefly let up and the three of us lie on the floor in the fading darkness, ears ringing, feet aching. Perhaps every party should be held in a tent in the middle of nowhere—you have to commit that way; there's no sloping off after half an hour. The Banjo Player dozes, and our chat meanders round to the subject of New York.

"Why don't you just move there for good? Why go to so much trouble for a few months?" N asks.

"Ha!" I say, but he's waiting for more. "Visas, mainly—boring red-tape stuff."

Beyond the window, a washed-out dawn is creeping up on the sleeping countryside, illuminating the fields, mist-drenched and milky green.

"Visas," he echoes, mulling it over until a thought strikes him. "I have a green card—that's halfway to an American passport. Wanna get married?"

"Ha!" I say again. Then, "Okay."

"Ha!" says the Banjo Player, who turns out to have been awake all along.

Yes, N is joking and so am I, but the funniest part is that until I embraced chastity, I'd not received even a joke marriage proposal. Surely this was progress. How proud of me all those chaste comportment manuals would be!

The next day, on the way to the train station, I find myself almost telling N about my quest. "I'm having a year of change," I say, stopping short. "I'm having one of those," he replies. Neither of us elaborates and we sit in silence for a few minutes as the hills splash by. N explains that a few years ago, a friend of his brother's came to stay at the rectory. "I drove him to the same station I'm taking you to, and his whole life changed on the platform. He had this epiphany. When he went back to the city, he quit his job and bought a dairy farm. He makes artisanal cheeses now—wins awards for them."

We miss my train by minutes. "I'm telling you, it's Epiphany Central," he says excitedly, handing me my bag with an unconvincing assurance that another train will be along soon. Planting a quick kiss on my cheek, he turns and is gone. Up and down the deserted platform of Epiphany Central I pace, pondering the events of the past forty-eight hours and considering my feelings for N. I stop right there—my feelings for N? Now that I am out of his orbit, the very idea seems ridiculous. Never mind that he is so radically not my type; I am clearly not his, either, considering that we seem to be back at square one again. As a prelude to his dashing off just now, he suggested that we go for a drink when he passes through London on his way back to New York. He has no idea of when this will be, because he has some thinking of his own to do. As the sun dived behind a thick cloud, his vagueness fogged the progress that I thought we'd made.

When I embarked upon this strange quest, I knew only that I needed to—I had but the haziest idea of why. I thought it had to do with my relationships, and, in particular, my relationship with sex, yet from here I can see that my dissatisfaction was more widespread: it was an entire way of life that I'd grown tired of. I'd decided that I wanted to stagger off the emotional roller coaster of sex, without for a minute imagining that chastity would cause a whole lot more up-heaval, leaving me stranded in the middle of the West Country, shivering as I wait for my epiphany to pull in.

Eventually, I give up on revelation and pin my longing on the arrival of the train—perhaps it'll have a tea trolley, maybe even a packet of those nice currant biscuits. The heavens are still gray but sunbursts strike the green, green hills, throwing the scene into hyperreality. It's beautiful. What's more, being marooned on the platform is oddly restful. A train will turn up eventually, so I'm not stranded, but I am in the middle of nowhere. There's nothing to do, no one to see, no place to wander. The reception on my BlackBerry comes and goes too whimsically for even an e-mail to slip through.

Is this my epiphany? That sometimes, just standing still for a moment, staying put and committing to a place, can bring peace? This thought, in turn, leads me back to N. What would it be like to stay in one place with him? To settle down? Finally sitting on the train, I take one last look at the station as we pull away. It's then that I see it: here in the sleepy back-of-beyond, a billboard advertising trips to New York.

The rest of June passes in a blur of preparation, of planning and re-planning. A family housing crisis throws everything into perspective, making my chaste challenge seem at once less and more important. Meanwhile, I have filled an entire room with taped-up boxes, each bearing a number that corresponds to a careful list, though really it's all just stuff—so much stuff. What makes it seem extra strange is that most of the things that are truly valuable to me—work, photographs, music—fit onto a memory stick on my key ring.

At the end of the month, when I step out into a bleached summer dawn and haul my giant red suitcase toward a waiting cab, the only key jangling alongside it is the key to my storage locker. The traffic is still light, and as we speed across an overpass I look down and see the streets that lead to Jake's. The driver has the radio on, and it's at that exact moment that the minicab's incense-scented fug fills with a familiar song. It's Erma Franklin, begging her man one last time to take her heart, to break it. If this were a novel, I think—and then stop myself, because it isn't.

THIRTEEN

July OR Mirror, Mirror

A woman's chastity consists, like an onion,
of a series of coats.

—Nathaniel Hawthorne

As if I weren't already tiring of the self-examination that my vow has inspired, the first thing I see when I step into the apartment I'm calling home for the next few months is my reflection. The mirror is large and slightly foxed, so I look a little dusty round the edges. It hangs above a lacquered chest of drawers whose top is cluttered with silver-framed photographs. These are the second thing that I see, and they all feature a black cat with a white bib and socks.

In one transatlantic hop, I have become yet another single woman in Manhattan, and a cat owner, too. Sitter is the more correct term, because the feline in question comes with my sublet, but it's not a distinction that the stray hairs trimming my clothes are likely to convey. Visible only when I venture out, they lodge in hard-to-reach regions, peeking from hems and wriggling into seams, the international badge of spinsterhood.

Her name is Madame Butterfly, and if cats truly do have nine lives, she is on her tenth, at least. Her fur is still thick and sleek but the rest of her is roadkill skinny, her tail crooked. Her movements no longer recall the sinewy grace of her big-cat cousins, but are more birdlike—the hesitant, earthbound twitches of a creature accustomed to operating in another element altogether. Watch, and you'll notice that she appears to be navigating with her whiskers. This is because she is blind. She is also deaf, which accounts for the blood-curdling caterwauling that wakes me in the early hours of our first night together. If you can imagine a feline Hound of the Baskervilles, she is it.

Still, she's not in bad shape for a cat of twenty-one. While half of me regards her as a tragic freak of Upper East Side veterinary medicine and is unable to look at her for a full forty-eight hours, the other half applauds. Even in this ethereal state, she jumps. She may take a good half hour to shuffle into takeoff position, tentatively stretching out a paw to ascertain that the drop is where she thinks it is, and that drop may be only coffee-table height, but she still makes the leap, and she still lands on her feet, the essence of cattishness.

Madame Butterfly comes with some very specific instructions. She is supposed to be with me for only three weeks, at which point the apartment's owner will return from her cruise and take the cat upstate for the rest of the summer. But three weeks is a very long time when you're the equivalent of 102 years old and it's topping ninety degrees outside. If anything "happens," I've been told to wrap her bony little body in a towel and place it in the freezer. The fridge freezer in the kitchen, that is, not some great chest humming away in a far-off garage or basement. She would be stowed alongside the ice cubes and fat-free frozen yogurt. Whenever Madame and I coincide in the kitchen, I catch myself eyeing her dimensions, wondering: Could I do it? Would I do it? And should I fail, do I know any cat lovers in this city who might step up to the challenge?

I haven't seen N since he retreated across the bridge at Epiphany Central on that chilly Somerset afternoon, but he's tracked me down, and over a series of e-mails we hatch a plan: dinner, downtown, late. It is, I suspect, a date. To start with, some unnamed others were involved, but now it's just the two of us. Or rather, it's just me, because N is nowhere to be seen. Still, I'm glad to be indoors. It isn't hot, it's stewed and soupy—exactly the kind of weather I was warned about before committing to summering here. Leaving the air-conditioned apartment was like stepping into a sauna.

It's been a blurry ten days. I arrived just in time for Fourth of July celebrations, and that evening watched the fireworks from high up on a friend of a friend's balcony, my jet lag and the humid drizzle throwing a dreamlike veil across everything. As neon bloomed eerily in the indigo sky—a kind of mirror image of the cityscape spread out before us—we stood around drinking beer from Dixie cups.

Dixie cups!

I may be in a city I know well, whose secrets I've parlayed into trump cards in those laughably competitive conversations that we Brits like to have about Manhattan, but I'm also in a foreign country, and I feel it more with every passing day.

Back in the restaurant, which is Italian, I'm lingering at the far end of the bar. The waiters are fast and shouty—flirty, too, though I'm just beginning to feel in the way when I see a familiar figure shamble in.

I'm surprised at how strange his English accent sounds. In this symphony of glissando vowels and damped *t*'s, it is something we share. He is a prolific orderer, and the table is soon crowded with pizza, bread, pasta—everything good that is bad. We share all this, too. I have never seen N in his adoptive country, I realize, and as dishes come and go and glasses are topped up, I list the things about him that seem different here. First of all is the fact that we can, apparently, talk in New York City.

"So how are you?" I ask, and he tells me. He doesn't just say "fine"—in fact, he doesn't say "fine" at all; he confides that he's not so happy here these days, that he's thinking of clearing out of town, heading back to Austin, maybe, even returning to England. He liked being in his hilltop retreat, away from it all. Then he asks about me, and as I tell him—properly tell him—he listens. He may be less content, but he is also more relaxed. And, yes, as I steal glances at him, I can't help noticing that he looks fine—fine in the American sense of the word. He's torn the dry cleaner's cellophane from a fresh blue shirt, and it's bringing out his cornflower eyes.

It isn't just him, of course. I feel different, too. Despite having shared midnight drives through muddy countryside and shivered together in damp tents, despite our dinner beneath umbrellas, there is a first-date fizz to the evening. More than that, there is a frankness between us, a candor that is exhilarating. It's not physical in the way that my attraction to Jake was, but its effects are. I can feel myself sitting up straighter. My smile is growing brighter, our eye contact lasting longer.

Later that night, lying in bed and replaying it all—my own home movie flickering on the taupe walls of Madame Butterfly's apartment—I'll try to recall how being with N makes me feel. It's like doing something I've never done before, something faintly magical—finding myself riding a unicycle, say. This feeling of concentrated, quiet elation, as if I've been pedaling along and realize only as I stretch out my arms for balance that I'm managing it. Here I am, having dinner with a man I can tell everything to without worrying about what he thinks, a man I like who seems to like me back. Having already spent the weekend with him and his banjo-playing friend, we're now on a first date—it feels disconcertingly right. Of course, the one component that is still missing is sex, just as all those prim primers insist.

It's nearing midnight by the time we leave, reluctantly stepping out into an evening that is still airless and close. Standing on the pavement, we're suddenly gauche as we stumble through our fun-yes-again-soon-we-must's. His height makes me a little giddy, which might be why my farewell kiss lands on his mouth. Or maybe he moves a fraction to the right. But why am I trying to excuse this? Because it's quite nice—at least, I think it is, though just to be sure, that first kiss has already multiplied into another and another, each a question and an answer both.

I've been here before, kissing men on pavements. You've done it, too, I'm sure, and you, like me, may not always have meant it, not completely. Sometimes it's just too tempting or too awkward to resist. Sometimes you just don't know, so it seems only reasonable to try it and see. And at other times you're hoping against hope that a kiss will turn your frog into a prince, forgetting that when the princess puckered up, such a transformation was still unheard of: she kissed her little green friend out of love, pure and fairy-tale simple. But right now, right here, what am I doing?

"So you like me, then?" N asks, and just like that, he's called my bluff. He must doubt my answer, because he fills the second of silence that follows with words that I then replace with another kiss, leaning into him on tiptoes and momentarily letting myself go. On East Twentieth Street, right in front of the house where Teddy

Roosevelt, poster boy for the world's underdogs, began transform-
ing himself from a sickly asthmatic into the twenty-sixth president
of the United States, my most unlikely paramour and I embrace.

But what of his question—do I like him? I like him very much, of
course I do, but do I *like* him like him? Of that I'm less sure. My vow
has taught me that I need to be a little more cautious with my heart
along with the rest of my body. I don't want to grow too cautious,
but it seems okay that I've yet to develop definitive feelings for N,
even as the things about him that I *like* like are growing in number.
All are surprising, some more so than others.

Take this, for example. After the kiss, N walks me to a cab. We're
clumsy with desire and it feels like we're wading through water as
we cross one street and then another. He reaches for my hand and
then pulls me in to him instead, his arm slung around my shoulder,
his fingers pressing lightly on my neck. Leaning in to him is an un-
speakable relief, and it has to do with feeling small and surrender-
ing to someone bigger. These are deeply unfashionable feelings, and
yes, I'm uneasy about them, particularly as they recall some photos
I saw a few days ago.

They were taken by Dave, a sometime friend of my sister's from
art school, who decided that because I was in New York, I ought to
attend an art happening. It was in Harlem, and his beaten-up Cadil-
lac was starring. Hipster spectators milled around as a woman in
overalls fed a supersized section of plastic tubing through the open
windows of a line of vehicles, threading them together like rosary
beads. It took a long time, and then it was over.

With Dave's car released from its cultural service, we drove back
downtown, where he made me a gimlet and showed me around his
apartment, tactfully bypassing the bedroom. A parrot named Fred
Astaire hopped from rung to rung of a cage that he'd made from

9/11 debris. He'd made lots of the kitchen, too, and maybe it was the apartment's hand-fashioned quality that gave it a tree-house kind of feel. It was all very boy's own, until I spotted the series of photographs.

He'd taken them himself, and they showed Barbie dolls shot as if they were life-size models at work, at play, kicking back with the girls. The one I remember most vividly was a close-up, and it showed only Barbie's slender wrist and plastic hand, resting daintily on a thumb that looked like a giant's. It's that I'm thinking about as N closes the door to my cab and gives me a half-wave, half-salute, before heading toward the subway.

A few days later, I accompany N to a dinner party in Queens. Our hostess takes to the piano, and while we feast off chorizo and salted almonds in the garden, her bluesy riffs float out on night air that's lit by fireflies. This is only our second datelike date, and it's tough that it's such a public occasion, but should we each be quite so eager to talk to other people?

It's a smart, rowdy crowd, and among the eight of us, nine conversations seem to be running at once. I'm trying to listen to N, who is talking with extravagant enthusiasm about something that sounds interesting, if only I could stay tuned long enough to catch what it is. The conversation that I'm drawn back to again and again is at the other end of the table. A loud woman in fuchsia is describing some of the peccadilloes recently revealed across a dinner table a few blocks from here. My chaste ears are flapping, but it's her clincher that is so compelling.

"And then they turned to my husband, and he said, well, I like to be *inside*. It shocked them!" It's tempting to reveal my own shocking sexual status, but the conversation rushes on while I'm still mulling it over. It's right that I stayed quiet, I decide: chastity has returned to me a sense of the private, of an inner space that is mine and mine alone. There's also the fact that it's a conversation I've yet to have with N.

Afterward, we share a cab back to the island and I ask him up to meet Madame Butterfly, he being a cat lover. His stroking doesn't win much of a reaction, though I'm watching closely. You can tell a lot about a man by the way he strokes a cat, someone once told me. We end up sipping bourbon on the sofa together. It hasn't seemed a large sofa when it's just been me and my books, but there is so much space between us, I'm forced to rethink. N stretches and sighs, sweat beading on his brow as he clears his throat once, twice. "I don't know how to play this," he says.

"This?"

"You."

"Play?" Did I say we two were able to connect conversationally here? I might have been wrong.

"I'd just like to move beyond the awkwardness."

I think about this a moment. Moving beyond the awkwardness has usually meant going to bed. Just now, for instance, I tried to kiss him as a way of ending that ridiculous dialogue. Sex is a great short-cut to intimacy, but intimacy arrived at that way hasn't lasted for me, not in the past. I'm casting around for the words to explain this—for an opener to the conversation that I really should have with him—when N decides to claim that kiss after all. Even with the air-conditioning chugging away, it's so hot that he is actually dripping sweat, and this turns out to be a novel kind of icebreaker.

A short while later, he undoes our hot tangle, hauling himself up from the sofa, a little less awkward now. He holds out his hand and I take it, allowing him to lead me through my own apartment to the bedroom.

"I don't know," I say as he gestures toward the bed. "It's very . . . catty. I wouldn't want to move her," I add, nodding to Madame, curled up on her side, looking almost sprightly in her sleep. It's not that I've suddenly become a cat person, but I am playing for time and putting off my real explanation.

He pauses to consider her, this man who claims to like cats so much, then, shrugging, says: "She's blind and deaf—the perfect witness." Carefully avoiding her, he lays me down across the other side of the bed. For a long minute or two, we look each other squarely in the eye—a searching, serious look, each sizing up the other.

"I think it's time for me to go. You understand, don't you?" And with that, he breaks away his blue gaze and pads through into the other room and out of the apartment. The awkwardness has gone and so has he. Do I understand? I look over at Madame B for help. Her ear twitches, but she seems pretty clueless, like he said. It's just the two of us now, she on her side of the bed, me on mine.

The explanation is a few days coming. We're meeting for after-work drinks and I'm running very, very late, but I really am running, despite the usual heat. In the right mood, this is a city where things seem perpetually on the up. Construction is everywhere—offices, hotels, gazillion-dollar condos. Half the time you're walking beneath the noisy shade of scaffolding. But in the wrong mood, everything seems to be coming down. Those same construction workers are demolishing, the sidewalks are cracked, the tarmac is melting. On this particular evening, there's the added confusion of roads still closed after an underground pipe exploded twenty-four hours earlier, sending a geyser of steam and mud roaring forth down near Grand Central, just around the corner from where I'm headed.

It's been a long, long day and I'm so screen-dazed that my eyes have forgotten how to blink. Spinning through revolving doors into the icy cool of the bar, I stride straight past N, who's tucked away in a leafy nook. He calls out as I charge by again, pulling over an armchair and ordering me a martini.

Gazing across at him, I see a man who is Jake's polar opposite, the one so silky smooth that I slid right off him, the other—N— almost porous. A person who swelters in the swelter, he soaks me up, feeling everything that I feel, even my doubts about us. I owe it to him to explain the drawing back that we both sense—I owe it to him to explain my vow.

The story that I've been telling you over all these pages isn't a simple one to condense. Whenever I've tried to yell snatches of it across social dins, filleting it for friends or finessing for would-be lovers, it has ended up mangled. I tell them what it isn't. Or I insist that it's fluffy—why, it's almost pink! And I blush. This time, it's easy. That surprises me, but not as much as N's response. He doesn't laugh. He doesn't shy away. Instead, he orders us another round of martinis and tells me a story of his own, one that very nearly says "Snap!"

At around about the time his twenties blurred into his thirties and his university years began receding into nostalgia, he realized that something had gone wrong. Not that his lifestyle wasn't enviable—as a tall, blue-eyed, very British Brit with an intense, offbeat charm, never mind his rock credentials, an ever-younger procession of Manhattan women passed through his life, some offering their hearts as well as their immaculately groomed bodies. Still, it had become boring, and earlier this year, he tells me, he'd decided to stop, to take a good look around him and, if necessary, wait a while for something more meaningful to come along. He doesn't use the word *chaste,* but nor does he flinch when I use it.

"You and me," he now says. "We're more than friends, you'd say?"

After all those twentysomething relationships in which I was craving clarification, a definition, I'm now being offered the chance to pin a word to what is going on, and I can't. Nor can N, not to his satisfaction. But the more I think about it, the more I find myself resisting the idea. This year of chastity has taught me many things about relationships, but it has also taught me how to be alone. I'd always thought that was something I was good at, but I now see that so much of my energy back then was spent in pursuit—of things, ideas and, yes, men. Without sex, my relationships are at once less complicated and more complex. I don't know if I'm ready to sacrifice that just yet.

My life in this city has become all about speed, at least on its shook-up surface. I tear from place to place, enslaved to a diary that begins at around six A.M., when I'm already behind on European time, and stretches late into the night, liquid and unplanned. It's Manhattan's smallness that makes such a sprawling schedule possible.

At either end of the candle, I glimpse the city's secret self: the fruit cart that sets up for business at three A.M. and is bafflingly gone by the time the rush hour commences, or, a few hours later, the girl—fancy-frocked with shiny blond hair—walking in flip-flops up Lexington Avenue, a smile on her face and the ribbon ties of a pair of satin shoes spilling from her hands.

That girl made me feel nostalgic. I love it, this whirl I've been caught up in since I arrived, but it isn't something I'd choose if I were here indefinitely. Being in a city on a three-month trial is a very present-tense experience, and though I'm relishing it, I'm not quite as enthralled by it all as I would have been a year ago—or ten years ago, back when I was around about the same age as that girl, with my twenties stretched out ahead of me like a yellow-brick road.

My vow of chastity has thrown into brassy relief some of my life's other less chaste aspects, making me at once more appreciative and less desirous. It isn't about excess—I haven't been hiding a trophy wife's shopping habit or a reality TV contestant's partying from you—but it does have something to do with tone. The Scottish philosopher John Macmurray arrived at an intriguingly broad definition of chastity. Writing in 1935, he knew that plenty of his readers still craved a flat condemnation of premarital sex. He refused to give it to them. Instead, he elaborated in *Reason and Emotion* on his notion that "chastity is emotional sincerity."

"Honesty is expressing what you think, chastity is expressing what you feel," he explained. It's about being true to yourself and frank about what it is that you want. A social rule was no substitute—only emotional integrity could empower a person to differentiate between "mutual want" and true love, to resist "self-deception in the face of desire." There it is again—desire in all its come-hither finery. Macmurray was a Quaker, but rather than invoke the usual hellfire and damnation as punishment, he conjures up a strikingly modern scenario.

"In all enjoyment there is a choice between enjoying the other and enjoying yourself through the instrumentality of the other," he cautions, the first scenario being love, the second lust. And even when it's mutual, pure unadulterated lust doesn't lead anywhere good. Two people who tumble into bed together in such a way "do not meet as persons at all; their reality is lost. They meet as ghosts of themselves and their pleasure is a ghostly pleasure that cannot begin to satisfy a human soul, and which only vitiates its capacity for reality."

What makes his interpretation of chastity extra intriguing is that a work of art, a film or a book—a lifestyle, even—could all accordingly be described as either "chaste" or "unchaste." Without knowing about Macmurray's ideas until now, I've been stumbling toward a similar definition. Along the way, I've discovered a quietness, and it's this that stops me from falling completely for the city's surface fizzle. When Shere Hite compiled her 1987 study *Women and Love,* she drew on the responses of thousands of anonymous questionnaires. This is what one woman said about life without sex: "What is lacking in intensity allows space and clarity—an ink-and-brush drawing of an iris, as compared with Van Gogh's vivid oil painting." It's what I mean by quietness. Of course, New York City itself is more like a Jackson Pollock, but my ink-and-brush iris has found a corner in which to bloom, slightly out of season.

On the eve of the anniversary of my last official sex, I find myself in another cab with N, stuck in traffic. We've been to Queens again, this time for a barbecue with old friends of his, meeting early in a bar where the scene doesn't get going till late. There was a baffling choice of seats—armchairs, leather cubes, the kind of stools that make you slouch unless you assume a sufficiently look-at-me posture. There were tables set off to the sides, sofas and tucked-away booths. And there, right in the middle of the room, was a large, velvet, raspberry-colored mattress. We both tried very hard not to see it as we made for a booth.

Our kisses aren't yet taken for granted. We still haven't quite made up our minds about each other, and my vow has given us more space than usual. Pulling back to look at N, I wonder whether his is a face I could look at forever. It's certainly not the one I'd imagined, but perhaps that's a good thing. There he is, with his curls and his lean wit. Without my vow, I would have written him off.

We all have types and mine is generic but fiercely clung to: dark-haired, olive-skinned, not short but never tall, whatever they themselves say. N is someone else's type. He is Nordic in coloring and stature—not freakishly tall, but easy to spot in almost any crowded room. I know that because in spite of those anomalies, he's become someone I seek out, someone close. Thanks to my vow of chastity, I've given him time and given us a chance. This man I wouldn't have taken into my bed is edging his way into my heart.

FOURTEEN

August OR *What a Woman Wants*

We are always inhaling at the same moment
and we are always exhaling at the same
moment. It is very intimate, but it is not the
kind of intimacy people are used to.

— Christie McNally, Buddhist teacher*

"**W**hat do you want?" It's the question that I hear more than any other in New York. Every lunchtime, it flies at me across the salad counter at the deli. From the far end of the line I try to prepare for it, wondering whether tuna with sun-dried tomatoes and fresh peas might be inspired or inedible, rolling the words in my mouth as if their letters might yield a flavorsome clue. Maybe I should ditch the tuna in favor of feta, or perhaps tofu, though it's so beige and wobbly-looking.

But it's no good. The three men behind the counter are scoop-chop-tossing at such hypnotic velocity that already I'm up. Stymied

---

*Christie McNally enjoys a chaste union with Michael Roach. In ten years, they haven't been more than fifteen feet apart; they eat from the same plate, read the same book simultaneously and do yoga together, breath for breath. They have never had sex.

by choice, I name the brightest ingredients, the ones whose pronun-
ciation is least likely to cause confusion and, heaven forbid, slow
things down (tomato went ages ago).

"Red pepper, sweet corn, broccoli and . . . tuna. Please." But even
then I'm not in the clear.

"Chopped?"

"No. Wait . . ."

"Ma'am?"

"Yes!"

"Dressing?"

"That one. Or . . ."

Too late. My red, yellow and tuna mush is now drenched in the
particularly nasty dressing that calls itself lemon and olive oil but
bears no relation to either, unless you count lemon-scented dish-
washing liquid.

What do you want? What-do-you-want? Whatdoyouwant?
Whenever I hear that question, I want to scream back: "What do I
want? I haven't had sex in twelve months! I don't know what I want!
I don't even know that sex is it anymore, but it's all I can think
about, so stop asking me about salad dressing or my career or my
heart. Please!"

N's voice has joined those of my interrogators. It's quietly be-
seeching as we lounge in a succession of bars shivery with air-conditioning. Even the ice seems extra cold in these places, clinking heavy
in the bottom of my drained tumbler and turning my breath to mist
as I stretch out my tongue for a last drop of fiery bourbon, stalling
to think of an answer that is true.

What *do* I want?

From N, the question is loudest when he doesn't voice it at all.
Like the other night, for instance, as we sat in a cab on the Brooklyn

Bridge, stuck in traffic and moving absolutely nowhere. Trapped, with water on either side and a long line of umoving yellow stretching beyond and behind us, the passenger space suddenly seemed too tiny. To begin with, his head had been resting in my lap. Now he is hunched over, perspiration glistening on his temples as he sighs.

Work offers no respite. There, I hear it from my editor, who asks me repeatedly and with mounting suspicion. She doesn't quite understand why I'm here, and it bugs her. I've watched her interview people and it's uncanny—it takes just a few prosaic-seeming questions to prove that she knows more about her interviewees than they know about themselves. "I was feeling stuck in London," I tell her. "I wanted to shake things up a bit." The look on her face says that this is not only the wrong answer, it is no answer at all. I'm inclined to agree.

Want is something I've been wrestling with these past twelve months—the kind that can be sated and the kind that can't, the point at which it intersects with something more enduring, something like need or wish or love. In that context, I've figured out what I don't want, but I've yet to pin down what it is that I do want. And how does a person go about finding that out? Trial and error? Because that salad was a revolting combination.

Sex, you'd imagine, must be one thing that I absolutely want. Increasingly, my vow has been prompting concern. "Nearly there. Thank heavens—I've been worried about you!" a girlfriend fretted the other day. Everyone agrees that I must be longing for it to be over, and in some ways I am, but it's a very mixed kind of longing. I want sex, but only in the right circumstances. There was a moment back in April—back when I was caught up all over again in the Jake situation—when I'd have settled for far less, but resisting has made me stronger.

My lenient-seeming rules have encouraged this resistance, though not in the way you'd guess. Oh, masturbation relieves a certain kind of tension, but orgasms, it turns out, do not have a great deal to do with what I've been missing this past year. Enjoyed solo, they're ultimately as unsatisfactory as all the racy foreplay with Jake, and a poor substitute for penetrative sex. To think how comically unappealing that clinical term sounded at the start! I've since craved it erratically but insistently, a deep hunger that makes every euphemistic cliché ring true. But it's not that alone I'm looking for. It's a fuller, more multidimensional experience. And the longer I hold out, the more determined I become to wait for it.

Has my vow made me strong enough to implement all that I've learned, though? Of that I'm not sure, which is why I almost wish I had longer to go. My vow has become less of a nun's habit than a child's security blanket. It's something to cling to—a reason to say no. Saying "Oh, I'm on this crazy quest" is somehow a whole lot easier than explaining that you'd rather take things slower and get to know each other a little better—than explaining what it is you really want. My vow expires on August 12—perhaps I shouldn't be thinking of success in terms of whether or not I make it through these next few days, but of how I move on afterward. That, surely, will be the more meaningful test.

And how *will* I move on? I've thought plenty about deliverance day. I've focused so much longing on the date that in my mind it's become more talisman than reality. Lately, though, anxiety has infused the longing. What if sex is not at all like riding a bicycle—what if it can be forgotten? Over the centuries, a prominent strand of Christian thought has claimed that we cannot ever forget Adam and Eve's knowledge—the original sin that got us kicked out of paradise and has stained humankind ever since. Will it really feel like losing my virginity all over again? Because that is what's implied by those who speak in terms of "revirginization." Periodically popular among jaded celebrities and born-again zealots alike, the notion has been given new weight in recent years by the rising number of predominantly Muslim women who opt for vaginoplasty, making their wedding night one of agonizing pain. This seems to be going back in all the wrong ways.

Going without cannot take us back, but it can take us forward in a new direction. While sex can make you feel at one with your body and the world like nothing else, not having sex connects you to your body in a different way. During the course of this year, in the quieter moments—of which there have been many, though I may not have always written about them here—I've become attuned to other needs: the longing for true intimacy, the desire for a connection capable of enduring across distance and time, an aching loneliness that has nothing to do with sex, because it's gripped me in the past with another sleeping just inches away. All these wishes feel acutely physical, which is perhaps why I've tended to confuse them with sexual urges. Sex did dull them—or it appeared to, but afterward, it would turn out only to have sharpened them.

While closing myself off physically, I've opened up more psychologically. Though I haven't always dressed in a strictly chaste fashion, I've achieved the cocooning that had felt so necessary at the start of the year, and that has given me a safe place from which to reach out in a more daring, less guarded way than when I'd put myself physically "out there."

At times, I've even felt as if my body were undergoing a second puberty. Germaine Greer is often quoted as asking this: "If a woman never lets herself go, how will she ever know how far she might have got? If she never takes off her high-heeled shoes, how will she ever know how far she could walk or how fast she could run?" I charge along in heels and that hasn't changed, but I have let myself go. I've left my legs unwaxed and I haven't bothered to shave my armpits, and beneath it all, my relationship to my body has subtly changed— it feels more my own. In a strange, wholly unexpected way, it also feels—well, sexier.

It took a recent episode for me to appreciate it. The nicest dress I own is the dress I wore to be Victoria's bridesmaid. Most brides put their friends in such bizarre outfits that they can never be worn again; mine was too nice to wear again, and it showed up the rest of my wardrobe something rotten. She gave us each an enormous budget and carte blanche—as long as our chosen dress wasn't black or patterned, anything went. That makes it sound like a dreamy shopping assignment, but I must have tried on almost every dress in London that spring. What I finally found was a halter-necked sheath in gathered yellow-gold satin. Though it was sleeveless and plunged—at the back— it wasn't exactly sexy (picking a sexy dress would have been breaking the biggest bridesmaid rule of all), and yet it required a certain sexual confidence to carry it off; otherwise it looked like a sack. And a sack is a sack, even when it's stitched from such beautiful cloth.

I bought it in the middle of my first dalliance with Jake. I've tried to wear it so many times since, but when I slip it over my head and venture a look in the mirror, I see a girl in a sack. A couple of days ago, that changed. I've lately got to know a real New York character, a sixtysomething dandy who seems to have been in all the right places at all the right times. Right now, he's in a palatial rent-controlled penthouse just a few minutes' stroll from my sublet, and from there he occasionally issues intriguing invitations: lunch in the vegan restaurant where he dines every day in the same booth; a brunch for a cast of A-listers whose names he is far too discreet to use in full; or, on this particular early evening, just a glass of something cool high up on his terrace. Afterward I'm off to the opera—the Chinese opera—thanks to a colleague with a spare press ticket. Actually, I've doubts about the opera, but if nothing else, it seems like a good opportunity to dress up. Should I try that dress one more time? Its folds of heavy fabric give me a shiver of sheer delight as they ripple down over my body. When I glance in the mirror, it doesn't look at all sacklike—which is lucky, because I'm running late. I don't have time to dry my hair, but as I dash those few blocks, not even wet locks dress this dress down. It being New York City, though, no one gives me a second glance, and I don't need them to, either: possibly for the first time ever, I've no use for the validation of a stranger's appraising gaze.

These triumphs make me all the warier of my vow's imminent expiration. One of the many arguments against chastity is that it whips people up into such a frenzy that it skews their decision making; that with sex pressing so hard on their minds, they become unable to see past animal attraction. Does this mean I need to decide in advance what I want, lest I'm seized by desire on the stroke of midnight and throw myself into the nearest willing arms? And there it is again, that question.

If you'd asked me just a week ago whose arms they might be, I'd have said N's—I'd have said his name and then thought about it a second, a secret smile playing on my lips as I imagined how it might be, because, yes, I've had decidedly unchaste thoughts about him. He's thought about it, too—he told me as much. "Do you mind?" he asked. I didn't mind. Instead, I chalked it up as another of the pleasures we cheat ourselves of in our sybaritic haste.

But I've also been thinking about him in other, less X-rated ways. Last week, I was chatting with a new friend, Jessica. She is edging toward her midthirties—an ultrasuccessful cookery writer blessed with charm and a quietly original way of thinking. She also happens to be single. "Actually, it's worse than that," she said, sighing, over tea and home-baked madeleines. "There are no more men in my life that I wonder about. This'll sound crass, but you know—the kind who fill your sort of mental wet dreams." I do know, I think. She means those men whose potential you fall asleep on each night. The precise scenarios may be tame or steamy, but it's our hopes that lend them their charge—boundless future-tense visions of togetherness. Female sexuality is so much more nebulous than men's. Having been extrasensitized to my own this past year, I can also testify that it ebbs and flows in mysterious ways. We women can fake an orgasm—what man can do that? And while female arousal has its telltale indicators, none is as clear as men's. When I think about it, some of my most erotic memories aren't to do with sex per se, but sex recollected. It's almost as if they are memories of memories.

Take this one, for instance: it's five years or so ago and I'm breakfasting with a guy I liked on and off—a guy who seemed to like me back, though we never quite coincided in our ons and offs. We're sitting in a coffee shop full of Saturday bustle. Before us are giant mugs and muffins, balanced precariously on a table crammed with fat weekend papers. When a supplement slithers to the floor, I bend down to pick it up, and as my hand touches its shiny cover, I feel his hand on the base of my back, just there in the gap between my T-shirt and jeans. Skin on skin, cool but not cold. It was a gesture so much more lingeringly erotic than the kisses we'd snatched on night buses or the way I'd woken to find him clinging tightly to me—too tightly, a desperate, impersonal hug that made me wonder to what dark place his dreams had taken him.

For me—and for many of the women I've spoken to, whether as

friends or while researching some article or other—a large portion of sex is in the mind. In 1992, sexologist and G-spot expert Beverly Whipple joined forces with her Rutgers University colleague, neuroscientist Barry Komisaruk. Together, they measured the heart rate, pupil dilation, perspiration and pain threshold of human guinea pigs, reaching the fascinating conclusion that some women can actually *think* themselves to orgasm. (Coupled with evolutionary psychology, this might explain more recent research that shows women experience more orgasms with rich men.)

This brings me to a confession: N is no longer the only man on *my* mind. While New York's foreignness is still creeping up on me—the longer I spend in this city I thought I knew, the more it feels like abroad—in other ways I'm beginning to live a little less like a tourist.

I've begun taking my tea iced. I've garnered nail-bar recommendations and acquired firm opinions on which route my cab driver should take from the Upper East Side down to the West Village, say. I've even seen my first rat—scuttling between two pieces of prime real estate on a thunderous evening when clouds hung low enough to snag the tops of the tallest buildings. Now I've been initiated into one of the city's most arcane rituals: the blind date.

An older work friend here set me up with one of her younger cousins. Though not yet forty, he runs his own private equity firm. He also buys art and reads books—not dry management tomes but novels, essays, poetry. How could I resist? After all, this is the home of the date, and when in New York, do as the New Yorkers do, right?

Need I mention that I Googled him before agreeing to the date? My search conjured up pictures of a face that was generically handsome, completely confident-looking. His eyes were gray, his smile open and his thick hair cut on the long side for a man in his line of business, suggestive of a yen to escape. For the occasion, I chose a dress whose full skirt met an empire waistline with a big-bowed sash—prim, though, as I couldn't help noticing when I passed a shiny shop window, it also made me look like a giant present. Bursting late, as usual, into the club's air-conditioned cool, I found myself looking straight into that same face, watching something lovely happen: both of us realizing that we'd hit upon that rare thing, a blind date with a person we might actually have picked out for ourselves.

That first date was perfect in its way. He named a place that I'd avoided until then—the sister branch of the latest London media spot to open Stateside. The choice of venue had made me doubtful—too obvious, too much a part of what I've been trying to edge away from this year—but his explanation was winning: he'd thought I might be feeling homesick.

The place turned out to be a lot smaller in reality than it looks on-screen, and a lot friendlier than the London original. We sat up on the roof, with electric views shimmering all around us. Like all perfect faces, Mr. Date's has a tiny flaw—an almost unnoticeable scar above his left eyebrow—and it was oddly entrancing as I listened to him tell me about his favorite writers and artists. Though we differed on the first, we soon found a photographer we both loved. And then suddenly it was time to leave—I was headed back uptown, a kiss on my cheek and curiosity in my heart.

The next morning brought a flawlessly romantic e-mail, informing me that he'd have been happy to talk all night. Could we meet again on Monday? Mr. Date also added another invitation—a visit to an art gallery upstate, which doesn't reopen until September. What is so appealing about him is his certainty, his complete confidence in the future.

Certainty is something we all crave in relationships. Take the cocktail writer I met a few weeks ago. Precociously pedantic when it comes to booze, he's still in his twenties—just young enough for his faint swagger to seem charming, like a sign of youthful self-protection. One evening, I'm at a bar with him, gingerly sipping something called a Dreamy Dorini Smoking Martini while he explains his rule of dating.

"It's my rule of three," he says. "You kiss within the first three dates, have sex within the first three weeks, and say 'I love you' before three months are up. Fail to accomplish any of them within the allotted time, and the relationship will fail—there's no point carrying on, you've got to get out quick."

A while ago, I'd have thought it sounded cynical. It does, but the cynicism is only a ruse. Beneath it is an urge to protect, to comprehend, to codify. It's part of the same urge that made me give up sex for a year, hoping I could find a way of hunting for love without getting hurt. What gives the game away is the number he limits everything by. Three belongs in the realm of make-believe—it's the number of little pigs, of bears and wishes.

It's also the hour at which we finally leave the bar and I head home to fall instantly asleep, completely missing a tornado—the strongest ever to hit New York City—that touches down just across the river in Brooklyn. The next morning my head is pounding and the city is deluged. Flooding has closed large tracts of the subway and the buses are overcrowded, stuck in streets whose gutters have become streams.

Around lunchtime, I realize I'm supposed to go to N's for dinner. He hasn't yet let me see his apartment, and this seems a bigger deal than his offer to cook for me. Still, I'm tempted to cancel—behind with work, faintly hungover, and not even sure I'll be able to get downtown. Then, just like that, the sun comes out, and within hours everything is back to normal. Everything but my head.

Maybe it's my migrainous way of seeing that makes N look differ-ent when he opens the door. He has just stepped from the shower and is buttoning up a fresh shirt as he kisses me hello and lets me into an apartment flooded with evening light. The effect is so uplift-ing that I don't notice the scores of books or the tangle of amplifiers.

Later, after we've eaten and talked and talked some more, he puts on a country-music album, and as we lie there, arms wrapped around each other, baby-voiced women and melodious men sing sto-ries of trucks and grocery bills, of heartache and the sweet trials of day-to-day loving.

We drift off like that, and it's gone midnight by the time we wake. N asks me to stay but I shake my head. With my year due to end just days from now, the coziness seems even more of a threat than all the torrid emotion that Jake and I stirred up together. There's also the fact that earlier, as my eyes had slid over his book-shelf, they'd alighted on a spine bearing a one-word title, big enough to be read from across the room. *Doubt,* the book was called.

New York rubric doesn't assume exclusivity until you've had "the conversation." N and I have had many conversations, but not that one. This doesn't stop me from feeling guilty, and feeling guilty doesn't stop me from looking forward to a second outing with Mr. Date. We're more lenient with ourselves when we're abroad—more prone to self-indulgence or trying something different—and in a strange way, my chaste endeavor has made the whole of my life feel like a foreign country.

Mr. Date suggests dinner at one of those neighborhood places so good the locals keep it to themselves. It's a Japanese restaurant, and the decorum and ceremony with which everything is served fans the spark I'd felt over drinks. Nightcaps on another rooftop bar fol-low, with the merest hint of a breeze stirring the sultry August air as the hands of the clock slide into the early hours. He compliments my earlobes, which seems hilarious and yet immensely touching— no one has ever done that before. In the elevator, we kiss.

"I've been wanting to do that all week," he whispers, and though I'm woozy with enchantment—his gray eyes, the citrus tang of his olive skin, the way he has access to all the city's high places—I can't help thinking that a week doesn't sound so very long.

When the stroke of midnight ushers in August 12, the end of my self-imposed drought, I'm catching up with Jessica and a couple of her girlfriends—equally impressive, dauntingly well-groomed women. By the time I arrive, they've already reached the bit of the evening where the talk is about men. It has a tart edge, and reminds me of all that I'd been hoping to avoid when I began this year. I don't blame them—their male counterparts seem just as judgmen- tal, just as demanding—but nor do I want to become them.

This stops me from telling them about my vow, and though I wish I could have toasted its close with people who've been on this journey with me, I realize that I've mostly traveled solo. Back at the start, I'd imagined that The Group and Nina, my sister and mother, would all have played larger roles, but in truth, the vow has been isolating. Granted, I haven't felt as lonely as I've previously felt within relationships, but in some ways it has kept me locked in with my own thoughts like a nun in her cell. I worry that her wimple, too, might have blinkered me.

With the liberating prospect of being able to look outward once more so close by, I can see that I might have strayed across the line from introspection to self-obsession this past year. My sister, for one, would agree. "It's not all about you," she'd snapped at me over the phone the other day. (That I'd already forgotten what it *was* about suggests she was quite right to do so.) But I can also see that before my vow—when it seemed to me that in obsessing ad nauseam about the men in my life, I was neglecting my own dreams and desires—this was its own form of self-obsession. Having been flattered into bed, I would from then on see men only in terms of their relationship to me. Female desire, psychologists say, necessarily contains elements of narcissism. While men want women, women want to be wanted. As Professor Marta Meana told Daniel Bergner in the *New York Times,* for us, "being desired is the orgasm." Art critic John Berger says something similar in his book *Ways of Seeing:* "Men look at women. Women watch themselves being looked at." If I'd been able to cast aside that prism, I might never have got involved with some of these men in the first place and that might have been preferable all round.

On my way home, I resist calling N or texting Mr. Date—after all, a full year hasn't quite passed. The day itself dawns cloudlessly blue. Before I've quite realized where I am in the calendar, I reach for my BlackBerry, which is flashing a long-programmed diary reminder at me: Jake's birthday. A year ago, a text to mark the same occasion sent me off on this surprising journey. Tapping out a brief greeting, I reflect on how fitting it is that the same should signal the start of its end, but when a reply arrives, I jump. I hadn't expected him to text back—and certainly not from my side of the Atlantic. He is safely on the other coast for now, but will be returning to London via New York.

In the months since I saw him last, I've given up thinking that I'll attain anything resembling closure with Jake. I've made peace with what passed between us. It was sex—nothing more, but nothing less, either. In its own terms, it was magnificent; it's just that those terms were not my terms.

N is due to head out of town on a three-week tour and has tentatively tried to persuade me to go with him. I did think about it, but
only for a second—after all the upheaval I caused getting myself to
New York, leaving seems ridiculous, and I'm not really a groupie.
We've arranged to meet for drinks later tonight, though, and it's all
I can think about as I sit alone in a radio studio, talking to callers-in
from another time zone.

Should the opportunity arise, I've decided not to sleep with N
tonight. Though it is very, very tempting, I don't want to do so
knowing that I won't see him for weeks. Yes, he could find love on
the road, but that's a risk I'd rather take. Among the past year's
many revelations, I've had to admit a certain passivity in my past
relationships. Making a choice to defer sleeping with N, then, seems
as positive a culmination to my year as sleeping with him. It's the
choice that counts.

Back on the airwaves, I notice that there are more callers-in than
usual. They don't really want to talk about books, either, but are
instead full of news of a meteor shower that is visible from both
there and here. I'd forgotten all about it because the meteors can't
actually be seen above Manhattan due to light pollution. Listening
to those other people trying to describe them, though, I can't resist
whispering the one adjective none of them uses: *orgasmic*.

Epilogue

Love is the answer but while you're waiting for
the answer, sex raises some good questions.

—Woody Allen

That's not the real ending, though, is it? I owe you a sex scene—I owed myself a sex scene. As it turned out, I was right to have felt trepidation about my year's end. If the journey I've been describing revealed how little I knew myself, its close showed me that in some respects I knew myself all too well. When presented with a choice, I would choose wrongly.

That evening, after the radio show and the drink, after I'd hugged N good-bye and wished him safe travels, I got into a cab and questioned the whole way home whether I'd made the right decision. Pushing open the door to the apartment, I stared hard at myself in that dusty mirror and nearly—so nearly—turned back there and then. What a great ending it would have made, meteors and all! But the mirror—and how bored I was of gazing into it—reflected something else back at me: on one level, I still wasn't sure about N, and meanwhile, there was Mr. Date.

Shortly afterward, Mr. Date invited me to the Hamptons—East Hampton—for the weekend, where he was throwing a party at his summer house. It was the prestige New York date and yet it felt ill-omened from the start. He called, wanting me to head out a day earlier, and when I told him that I had an immovable meeting and an overdue article to deliver before the weekend, an unseasonable coolness crept into his voice. Then I was struck down by a violent forty-eight-hour gastric flu. By the time Saturday rolled round, I was pale and fragile-feeling but bikini-thin. As I left the apartment, he called, and for a moment I thought he was going to put me off, but he was just checking that I was on my way.

He was a different person away from Manhattan—a person I didn't know and couldn't begin to talk to. The clapboard house was fronted by a pristine, fake-looking lawn. It was also full: colleagues, clients, old college buddies. The cast seemed to change by the minute, swelled by caterers and florists. After lunch, the two of us slipped away from the rowdy chaos and wandered down to a private beach. We lay side by side on the hot white sand while the roar of the ocean waves did something strange to sound, making the distance that was opening up between us seem even greater. Their crashing did nothing to muffle the insistent tap-tap-tap of a game of beach paddleball farther along the shore, nor Mr. Date's grumbling about it.

After so many perfect dates—too perfect, perhaps—it seemed I had disappointed him in some way. Every attempt at conversation drew us further apart. "Could you ever live out here?" he asked, gesturing to the dunes, the pretty painted houses. I mentioned something about the magic of being so close to the edge of land and he looked puzzled, talking instead of transport links. Had we been at cross-purposes all along?

The evening brought a dressy gathering and still more guests—brittle, strung-out girls and blogosphere princes who'd made virtual millions before turning thirty-five, but whose soft faces betrayed trust fund backing. There was something precarious about the scene, and it didn't just have to do with the jowly man tiptoeing along the pool edge, or the woman looking on and laughing a high, frenzied laugh. A photographer for a local zine slipped between groups, the glare of his flash like lightning in the dusk. I wanted to count the seconds in anticipation of thunder.

Later, the awkwardness intensified when it came to sleeping arrangements, which still hadn't been discussed. I think if I could just have found a way of telling Mr. Date where I'd traveled from, how I'd spent the past year, it would have been okay.

And yet, I couldn't.

All those months, all those lessons supposedly learned, and here I was, going to bed with a man who by that point felt like a stranger. How could this be happening?

There were no meteor showers over Long Island that night. The sex, predictably, was awful. Oh, there was jiggling and rubbing and rustling, and though he didn't show much interest in undressing me there was, eventually, full nudity. There was some friction, too—the wrong kind of friction. "You need to be more intentful," he huffed. Intentful? It seemed a word better suited to the boardroom. Could he have a secret corporate fetish? Perhaps I should offer to take minutes? I reapplied myself to the task at hand, but was fast beginning to feel like tabling a motion for dissolution. That was *all* I was feeling.

"One of the great glories of sex is the difficulty of talking about it—no other human activity, not even love, is so resistant to the assaults of language," wrote the critic Anthony Lane, articulating a truth universally acknowledged. Who'd have guessed that bad sex would prove most resistant of all? Suffice it to say, when it came, that moment I'd been denying myself for a full year, it was intensely, profoundly, unutterably anticlimactic.

My confidence was shaken—maybe I really had forgotten how to do this stuff? Mostly, I just felt ridiculous. What was the point of giving up sex only to repeat the exact same mistakes? Well, I had forgotten how to do something. Though I tried to put my heart into the performance, as once I'd have done, it refused to have anything to do with such a sham. Nobody in that bedroom was convinced. Getting into this situation suggested I'd made absolutely no progress, but my response showed just how much I had learned. I could tell the real thing from the fake, and from that there was no going back.

But I did have to get back to the city, and the sooner the better. On the bus, sunburned, embarrassed and, well, chastened, I gazed out at the ocean unsure whether to laugh or cry. The episode had been so awful it was comical, and yet didn't it make me an abject failure? Still, when a text from Jake popped up, I couldn't help laughing: another test that I was bound to fail? It was too absurd.

I beat myself up about the way my year ended, but from that moment on, things have been very different. We had a drink that evening, Jake and I, and together, we laughed some more about my weekend. It was good to see him. He was staying upstate and had to leave early, and that was good, too. For all its farcicality, the Hamptons episode was like one final mirror being held up to me: was that who I was? Possibly, but it was not who I'd become.

Traditionally, chastity has been a tool for transcendence, a way to slip free of both body and self, to sidestep the perceived confines of gender. For me, it ended up being the exact opposite. My twenties had created a disconnect between what I hoped for from sex and what the men in my life seemed willing to offer. I'd begun to doubt my own expectations, but those twelve chaste months reaffirmed my faith in romance, and taught me much else besides.

If you hold back physically, I learned, it makes it easier to open up emotionally. There are some conversations that you feel too vulnerable to have naked; slow the pace, and you'll find you can risk a little more candor—with yourself as well as with your partner. It takes the pressure off those bewitching early stages of a relationship, and yes, it helps sort the cads from the keepers. When it comes to courtship, the fly-by-nights lack the staying power.

It also taught me about emotional self-sufficiency. In a consumerist society, our desire is constantly being manipulated, and it's not simply our gastronomic, sartorial and cultural fancies that the billboards tweak; it's our more intimate hankerings, too. In tuning out those subtle and not-so-subtle come-ons, I've found within myself some of what I'd formerly looked to sex to provide. Ultimately, this makes relationships more fulfilling—you have more to offer, and you get back what you put in. Meanwhile, I felt its impact on other areas of my life, too, becoming more decisive and discovering fresh reserves of creative energy.

There were physical rewards as well. Heightened sensuality, for one—less really does become more. Scientists have proven that some women can think themselves to orgasm, but even the beginners among us can be thrilled through and through by a bright blue sky or a balmy breeze, by just opening our lungs and singing along to our iPods (not Erma Franklin's anthem but her sister Aretha's—the one about "Respect").

Curiously, while chastity deepened my understanding of love, it also gave me a newfound respect for its impish twin, lust. There's a store opposite the café where I sometimes go to work whose window is strung with tote bags. "True lust" reads one, its message emblazoned like a tattoo across a cherry-red heart. There is some truth there, but you don't really appreciate it until you try to resist it.

We've narrowed our definition of *sex* to a cartoonish hybrid, robbing ourselves of experiences and emotions; reintroducing the notion of chastity as an option broadens the erotic spectrum. We talk in terms of "sorbet sex" (an inter-course palate cleanser) and "cereal sex" (a one-night stand that leaves you hungrier than you started out). Compare that to "the heavy Mischiefs of vagrant Lusts" that *An Exhortation to Chastity* cautioned against in the eighteenth century. "Extinguish the smallest Sparks, lest they kindle the Fire of Lust in you" continues the tract, which ran through numerous editions over the course of fifty years. How much more tempting all that hectoring prochastity literature makes sex sound! Ironically, today's relationship best sellers are mostly aimed at rekindling that same fire, long since damped by permissiveness.

My chaste adventure highlighted other paradoxes, too. Sometimes, in trying to make the most of our unwanted single status—signing up for foreign language classes, committing to grueling exercise regimes, masterminding charitable initiatives—we become unapproachable. And then there's the pampering, the little morale-boosting treats—unchecked, they lead to the kind of self-centeredness that makes a person unable to compromise. As I've edged further into the decade that this book found me on the threshold of, I've watched single girlfriends fill their time so successfully with friends and family and work that their schedules simply can't accommodate another relationship. They've even formulated their own backup plans. Remember when the backup used to be the old friend you'd struck a pact with, to marry and start a family with if you both wound up still single at a certain age? As at least one movie is set to confirm, the twenty-first-century backup plan involves freezing your eggs for artificial insemination. It's a plan for one. Was my year just another example of this?

Me, myself, I—how I longed for a different pronoun by the time those twelve months were up. "We," for instance—that would do nicely. At the same time, I couldn't remember a time when I was more content to be single. Yet that year has enabled me to become part of a "we" thanks to conversations with women—and men—around the world who turned out to conduct their own personal lives along similar lines. They ranged from an Italian hotel receptionist in her early twenties to an L.A.-based actress in her late thirties, and even included an ex-marine. Many more have written, e-mailed or texted; their correspondence tends to be anonymous, underscoring another of chastity's perks: privacy.

Fads and fashion have an increasing influence in that most intimate sphere of our lives. Sex is becoming more and more of a performance. Never mind anxiety—never mind lighting and music. It's all about costumes and props, audiences even. The Web site IJustMade Love.com enables couples not only to log the time and place of their assignations, but to choose from five possible positions. Blame it on the Internet, blame it on porn—blame it, if you like, on Internet porn—but whatever the cause, this apparent need for external validation suggests that people are failing to fully inhabit their own most intimate experiences.

For me, chastity also revealed the extent to which our personal lives continue to be political. This seems especially true for single women, who attract more prurient interest than their bachelor brothers. The title of Helen Gurley Brown's iconic *Sex and the Single Girl* spelled it out as boldly as lipstick on the bathroom mirror back in 1962. No longer was the single girl to be treated "like a scarlet-fever victim, a misfit." Matched up with sex, if not Mr.

Right, she was to be rehabilitated as "the newest glamour girl of our times."

By the 1990s, when Bridget Jones tottered onto center stage, that sassy message of sexual entitlement had become enslaving. Singletons who weren't "shagging," in Bridget-speak, felt a level of lousiness completely disproportionate to their thwarted longings. Flash forward another decade, and there's *Sex and the City*'s Samantha Jones, rampaging through Manhattan's outnumbered men. Watch the early episodes carefully, though, and you'll hear a few telling asides that hint at a less perky backstory. Today, there seems to be no scope for such nuance. In the BBC miniseries *Personal Affairs* (2009), an archetypal Gurley Brown "glamour girl" offered some advice to a friend: The three things a girl can't live without? Two liters of water a day, a swish credit card and "healthy, regular, meaningless sex."

Our desire for, and right to, sex has been distorted into an enslaving necessity that has too many women making do, taking what they can get rather than holding out for what they might secretly yearn for: love. Yes, it works for some, but for the rest of us it can feel as if equal rights has morphed into the right to the exact same things that men have—subtly but profoundly different from giving us the right to the things that we as women need. And when it comes to sex, those needs tend not to be the same, despite ample overlap.

The study of female desire is a growing and fascinating field, though experts face a considerable challenge in disentangling nature and nurture. This is in itself instructive. As Meredith Chivers, a psychology professor from Ontario, told the *New York Times*, "So many cultures have quite strict codes governing female sexuality. If that sexuality is relatively passive, then why so many rules to control it? Why is it so frightening?" In a strange way, sexual liberation has become just another of those codes. Despite that movement's noble aims and undoubted gains, its legacy has made over female sexuality using all the worst tropes of masculine sexuality; it's depicted as predatory, unscrupulous, heartless.

The reality, meanwhile, is deeply conflicted. While sharply tailored women in TV dramas extol the virtues of clitoral collagen injections, others in real life lift their skirts for the surgeon and endure humiliating virginity tests or, if they've failed, vaginoplasty. We turn a blind eye to the fact that for many, virginity remains a life-or-death issue; that female circumcision means others will never know sexual satisfaction. At the same time, we pillory teenagers' abstinence pledges without pausing to consider how hard it must seem for them to plot a middle way. No wonder teenage girls are so enamored of vampires: those ethereally pale men are pure passion, yet they either keep their appetites in check or else behave with a courtliness that died out in living, breathing men eons ago.

For all that sex surrounds us, it remains a topic fraught with fear and anxiety—and ignorance, too. A girl may know how to give a professional-grade blow job, but she still may be clueless that the HPV vaccination, if she's had it, won't protect her from contracting throat cancer. And though it is men who carry the HPV virus, it is women who are being obliged to protect themselves—after all, boys will be boys, right? "Arm yourself for life," the slogan for a vaccine ad campaign, plastered over UK buses, tells teenage girls—an oddly combative metaphor suggesting that the gender wars may be forgotten, but they aren't yet over. Invariably, it's teenage girls who are on the frontline. In a tabloid world that ranks sexiness far above smarts and talent, it's little wonder that a place on the "slut list" has become a badge of honor among girls as young as fourteen in American high schools.

Last autumn, the UK's National Society for the Prevention of Cruelty to Children (NSPCC) released a survey that painted an even bleaker picture. One in six girls between the ages of thirteen and seventeen said they had been pressurized into sexual intercourse, while a quarter of those questioned had suffered some form of physical violence at their boyfriends' hands. Clearly, understanding that "no" means no is not the same as feeling you have the permission or the safety to say it in the first place. It's something that women twice the age of those girls can still feel. We've lost any sense of healthy emotional entitlement, leaving us with fewer and fewer reasons to say it. You're not in love? Even that isn't just cause when other polls reveal that plenty of younger men and women are having sex simply for the practice. The NSPCC survey revealed more distressing statistics: a third of those questioned said they had been sexually abused, and one in sixteen said they had been raped.

Would I say that I'm a feminist now? I would, yet during my chaste year, it sometimes felt that the lessons I was learning went directly against feminist rhetoric, pointing the way to a distinctly unevolved way of snaring a mate. That wasn't what my quest was about, of course, but I found it curious that the approach sometimes drew a sharp intake of breath from other women. Why is it so much more shocking to withhold sex in order to make a man love you than it is to go to bed with him, hoping against hope for the same outcome? Let's face it, neither tactic is wise.

Toward the end of my chaste year, an impressive New York feminist asked me whether I was "for or against" chastity. I felt browbeaten. Though we were eating brunch on a sun-splashed Sunday sidewalk, she seemed like someone who had time only for snappy absolutes, and that is part of the problem. What I'm for is reinstating chastity as an option, reclaiming it from the religious and political zealots who are so adamantly for or against. Chastity belongs back in the mainstream as a valid form of sexual expression, as a positive rather than a negative, defined not by what it declines but by what it bestows: romance, sensuality, emotional intimacy.

For some, chastity is inherently problematic, allied too closely to the notion that women want sex less than men. But here's the thing: most of us do want sex less than men—a certain kind of sex, that is. Plenty of men would rather not have that kind of sex, either. Yes, boys will be boys, but contemporary sexual mores short-change them, too. As the lead character in *Zack and Miri Make a Porno* (2008) protests in true mumblecore style, he was too scared to tell the woman he's slept with how he felt about her because they'd agreed not to let sex change them. "But it did. It changed me. That has to be love, right? That has to be love."

And what of love—did giving up sex bring me any closer? Well, I eventually got together with someone. The relationship didn't last, but it lasted longer that any had in a long while, and we both were serious about it from start to finish. Since then, there has been one more relationship. We turned out to share similar thoughts and stuck to the terms of my chaste year, admittedly helped along by frequent spells during which he was abroad. Still, I think it made the breakup easier and, more important, added something to our togetherness—not just spice, but tenderness. From one of those men I heard the words "I love you," and to the other I said them back. Not quite how it's supposed to happen, but it seemed like progress.

As I write this, two full years have passed since my chaste vow expired. If I tell you that I'm still single, will you sigh? Inasmuch as there was a questing element to my chaste endeavor, it was a quest to discover a fresh way of looking for love in the new decade I'd arrived in—my thirties. That, I've found. A good date now ends not with a "May I come in?" but with a "When can I see you again?" If it's accompanied by a lingering kiss laden with promise, all the better. I don't discount the fizz of physical attraction. In fact, I hope for it, but I do give it time to settle down a little, and that, too, can be fun, if not always easy. "To many, total abstinence is easier than moderation," St. Augustine quipped, and he was right. Unlike abstinence, chastity is an ongoing project. You can even be chaste within a sexual relationship. It insists on utmost honesty—with yourself, with others. Sometimes, that honesty is inconvenient. When a man who has been seductively whispering sweet nothings pauses to tell you that, by the way, he has no wish to get married again and the children he already has are enough for him—well, it's hard to recapture the mood. If those are things you truly desire, your only option is to turn his embrace into a friendly farewell.

But while there is less sex in my life, I'd gladly take any amount of accompanying frustration in lieu of the other kind—emotional frustration. The former passes, the latter persists. What there is infinitely more of these days is romance. Men have bought me dinner and flowers and silly, sweet gifts. They've strolled with me along beaches, met me at train stations, and paused for kisses beneath the dappled canopy of a towering oak. One even sent an old-fashioned love letter. Failing all else, they've called.

Each of these intrigues has seemed less ephemeral than many of the more physical relationships of my twenties, but something else has changed, too. These stories haven't become my life's defining drama in the way that they once would have been. Instead, I've spent some time living in Paris and bought a place beside the sea—a room of my own with the kind of fireplace you'd expect to find a mirror above, only you won't, not here. I've rekindled old friendships, learned to make perfect manhattans, and discovered that I enjoy gardening—in window boxes, at least.

Still, it's hard to shrug off the notion that in remaining single, I'm not somehow testifying to the failure of my chaste year. After all, books about single women invariably end up being about women who become part of a couple, who become *un*-single. It's a narrative pattern ingrained in us from our first fairy-tale reading, our first enraptured Disney viewing. The idea of a story in which the heroine winds up not merely single but contentedly so carries a dangerous frisson.

For this reason, I'm almost tempted to end right here, but that would be disingenuous. I can't give you wedding bells, but I will grant a peal of texts. It's the eve of the second anniversary of my chaste year ending, and I've left my seaside hideaway, bound for a London lunch with a long-ago lover who's running late.

His name is Jack, and though you haven't yet met him, he hovers in the background of plenty of the stories I've been telling. In some respects, he represents everything that I was rejecting when I chose chastity. We met at college, at a fancy dinner in one of those ancient, high-ceilinged halls lined with portraits of scholars and kings. His quick charm was compelling, and he had a mercurial brilliance. Afterward, I'd glimpse him around town—always running someplace, hot on the heels of some scheme or scam.

Our first real date wasn't until later, just after I'd broken up with the Pasha. We'd been to my favorite bar—the magical one, and now that I think about it, its magic stems in part from that evening. It had been snowing as we arrived, and by the time we left—late enough that even the doormen had gone off duty—the world beyond was transformed. The unsalted pavements were like glass, which gave us the perfect excuse to hold on to each other tightly. As we waited for a cab, we shared a smile, blinking away snowflakes. "Your eyes—gray or blue?" he'd asked. "Blue-gray," came my contrary reply—I couldn't help it; with him I was always myself. And then we kissed.

Other dates followed, each as flamboyant as the madly patterned shirts he wore. He'd arrive by rickshaw, or would take me someplace where the cocktails were served in pineapples. We'd turn up an hour and a half late for a Valentine's Day reservation and stay out until the whole city, it seemed, had gone to sleep. But beginning with that first kiss, each is a vivid memory, surprisingly undimmed by inebriation or the passing of time. What drove me insane was their complete lack of continuity. He'd text on Christmas Day, for instance, but in the silence that followed—months and months—its sweetness would acquire a generic ring, the kind of tipsy festive fondness you might send to half your phonebook. I almost didn't go to his thirtieth birthday party, having not seen him for about four months beforehand. I went in the end, which was lucky because it turned out to be an intimate black tie dinner whose seating plan placed me at his side. At the other end of the table, partially obscured by the miniature cherry orchard that formed its blossomy centerpiece, sat his parents. In between dates, I managed to live through complete affairs. Had I technically been cheating on him? I wondered as I sat beside him at that birthday dinner. I'd once joked that maybe we could see each other seasonally. We almost managed it.

After a few months of silence following his thirtieth, he called me as I headed home from dinner with Victoria. It was late, and he wanted me to jump in a cab and cross the city to visit him. Was I tempted? Oh, I was. But I knew a booty call when I heard one. I also knew panic, and that's what hummed on the line as he told me how he'd been out celebrating the engagement of yet another of his friends. Hearing him pleading was novel, but I was determined not to call that cab. We talked though—we talked and talked for hours. It didn't involve champagne or a mad dash to a ritzy restaurant. It didn't even involve being in the same zip code. But it was perhaps the best date we'd ever had.

If I were stretched out on a couch narrating this, it might be asked why Jack's name appears only now. It occurs to me that I was perhaps always hoping our story might become something else— one that didn't belong in any of the other chapters. The more straightforward reason is that we simply didn't have much to do with each other during my chaste year. When I glimpsed Dan and his fiancée ring shopping in Manhattan, I'd needed to get out of London to clear my head—and my heart—after yet another confusing episode with Jack (he'd cooked dinner for me and talked wildly of wanting children, then promptly gone to ground again). I returned to London, turned thirty, and met Jake. Jack moved abroad, changed jobs and met a girl who succeeded where I'd failed.

Months later, I was researching a magazine feature on casual sex. I'd sent round a plea to friends who might be willing to dish the dirt, and I had a particular question for Jack: had we been casual? Some weeks later came his reply: "I guess." My year without sex had begun by then, but a small part of me was still curious to find a label under which to file us away. Jack's response didn't seem definitive— there was something grudging in his assent, which left a chink of hope, were I looking for it.

By the time my year of chastity ended, his relationship had, too. In the tinsel-strewn wilderness between Christmas and New Year's, we'd met for dinner. It was unseasonably cold—storybook December weather, not the usual soggy grays of the English holiday season—but I couldn't help smiling as a text confirmed his lateness.

We hadn't seen each other in the four years since he moved abroad, but some things never change.

The neighborhood we'd chosen to meet in confirmed as much. Its stores sell classic, solid items made to last, inflated price tags their sole nod to modernity, and you can still find tucked-away bistros whose menus offer the same cassoulets and crème brûlées that they've been serving since the 1970s. Our reservation was in such a place. If you consult its *Zagat* entry, you'll find that it's recommended for romance and seniors. I hadn't, but I knew it as soon as Jack held open the door for me and we stepped into its plush, discreetly lit interior. It was too charming to be stuffy, and its seniority was of the intimidating kind. It made me feel as if we were kids still—uncertain. And that's the funny thing about the whole evening. Being with Jack had all the coziness of being with someone you've known for years and years, but there was something else, too—something new and shy. He still made me laugh, he still maneuvered his way recklessly around a menu—two of this, three of that, a bunch of those—and his smile could still set my heart somersaulting. At the same time, he'd become grounded. Though I couldn't quite figure out how his days were spent, he talked about his job with passion and humility. Here was someone I could respect, I realized, whose opinion mattered to me.

Courses came and went, I heard all about his new life in the Far East, and he had some questions about my chaste year. At one point, he glanced at his watch. I was still doing that early-hours radio phone-in, and had told him in advance that I'd need to leave before midnight in order to be home in time. "I just need to get to a landline," I hinted. What was I up to? Whatever it was, Jack wasn't about to collude in it.

Less than an hour later, I was in a cab, bound for the station.

We'd been so proper with each other, even our farewell kiss was without liberties. Our departure was so rushed, it took me a while to sense the disappointment underlying my astonishment. Had I ever been out with Jack and not gone home with him? The chaste me blushed to acknowledge it, but no, I had not. Had we both changed so much?

The next morning, in the cool light of the coming new year, all these questions were subsumed by a quiet delight: I'd gone home not with Jack but with a discovery—of a dear friend who'd been there all along, but whom I'd really glimpsed only that one time when we hung out on the phone. A few days later, he e-mailed, inviting me to visit him in the Far East. "I have a spare room," he wrote, "whatever that means."

We've stayed in touch since then, and though I haven't yet visited, we have talked dates. Now it's summer, and Jack is back in town—only briefly, but long enough for a long, long lunch. London is hot and still, its streets empty of locals. We'd hatched one of those plans that's doomed to chaos, and after fifteen minutes spent lost within a few blocks of each other—fifteen minutes that seem to sum up our fifteen years of knowing each other—we both make it to the same spot. He hugs me tightly before standing back to appraise me, and I take him in, too. His has a gleam about him, and though his shirt is a sensible stripe rather than a psychedelic paisley, he's carrying a large gift box tied with a bright orange ribbon. It's for me. Nestled inside is a set of chalky orbs. "Sex bombs," announces the label that Jack, too late, tells me not to read, rushing to explain them away as an impulse buy. They are supersized bath fizzers—a hilariously inappropriate token for any woman who aspires to sophistication, let alone chastity. But he's called my bluff, because later that evening, I'll dunk one in the tub, unleashing a torrent of pink and purple bubbles, and turning the water into a witch's cauldron. Who knew bathing alone could be such fun?

Over lunch, we talk about that dinner. "It completely threw me," Jack says. "You were running the show." This is news to me. What about my hints that I didn't technically need to get home, just to a decent phone line? He looks at me blankly.

Truthfully, I think we were jointly steering the course of that evening, and though its outcome irked me plenty at the time—I'd already served my year of chastity!—it affirmed all that I'd set out to prove at its start. In departing from our usual script, we've been jolted into another way of being with each other, one that's infinitely more rewarding, and more thrilling, too.

Unfortunately, it's got Jack thinking about chastity, too. He was so inspired by that evening and its unexpected end that now before he ventures out on a date, he chants a one-word mantra to himself: "chastened, chastened, chastened." I'm laughing as he tells me all this, but when he asks whether I'd recommend that he embark on a year of his own, I find myself trying to talk him down, just in case. "Maybe a chaste three months?"

To distract him, I ask a favor. A magazine needs a photograph of me with an ex—Jack sort of counts, and he's the only one I feel able to ask. Our waitress agrees to play photographer, and when I slip over to Jack's side of the table, he wraps an arm around my shoulders and pulls me in close. A short while later, I'll take a look at our waitress's handiwork and be struck by how happy we look, how disconcertingly right.

Too soon, our bill arrives. This time, we kiss properly. "So you'll come and visit?" Jack asks, and I nod before stepping reluctantly away. Back on that New York sidewalk, I'd wondered what would have happened if I'd called out, if my life had been a movie. I was right not to—I had no part in the story of Dan and his fiancée—but this is different. While life isn't a movie, least of all a romantic comedy, it can sometimes approximate one. After all, what could be more comically romantic—or should that be romantically comic?—than getting on a plane and traveling halfway round the world in order to try to seduce a man out of his chaste intentions? For now, I venture a last look back before turning the corner, just in time to see him watching me leave, a dazzled smile on his face to match my own.

Acknowledgments

Without stripping them of their fig leaves, I'm unable to thank the men who inadvertently inspired this book. For all the challenges of trying to be with them, I couldn't have done it without them. If they'll permit it, I offer a chaste peck on the cheek to each.

Of those I can name, the inimitable Elizabeth Sheinkman has been an inspiring supporter even before becoming my agent. She was this book's first champion out in the world, and, in particular, chaperoned it through the crucial early stages with stylish rigor.

My editor, Clara Farmer, and her stellar colleagues (Anna Crone, Juliet Brooke, Lisa Gooding and the focus group especially) at Chatto & Windus have provided rousing support and complete understanding from the very start. Clara's incisive thoughts have shaped the volume you now hold in your hands, and her wry marginalia kept me going in the later stages. Off the page, she has proven a source of unflappable grace—even when I turned up to lunch carrying a saw, even when the manuscript's delivery must in itself have begun to seem like a coy tease. In the U. S., Molly Stern, Kendra Harpster, the ever patient Amanda Brower, and the rest of the Viking team have dazzled with their commitment and professionalism.

Humble thanks to colleagues past and present at the *Daily Mail,* the *Observer,* Bloomberg and BBC Five Live, who provided encouragement and later—when the writing got under way and *in* the way of my journalistic commitments—indulgence.

Throughout, my mother has been my storytelling (and story-living) heroine, while my sister has been chief cheerleader (goading and vexing as only a dear sister can when that didn't work). I'd also like to thank my great-aunt for not asking these past months, as promised—and for having told so much over the years.

The storage key that I pocketed at the end of chapter 12 remained there far longer than I'd anticipated, and portions of this book I wrote as a nomad. During those months, family and friends were unfailingly generous with inflatable mattresses, desk space and, in some cases, entire houses. In particular, my gratitude to the great kindness of Gerry Fox in London, and Heski Bar-Isaac and Owen Sheers in New York. In Paris, James Linville scouted a dream writing apartment with a view of the Moulin Rouge's red glow and the city's best *tartes* on its doorstep. He also heads this next group.

To all the friends who so readily offered up enthusiasm, jokes and their reading time, thank you. In particular, for conversations timelier than they might have guessed, I'm grateful to Gavin Adda, Anthony Bale, Jonathan Coe, Eithne Farry, Gagan Grewal, Reva Seth, Hellena Taylor and Adam Thirwell.

Last, the following chaste treats kept me going, and are recommended to anyone who, by design or by accident, finds himself or herself wandering in the desert: pizza slices from Ben's, a cocktail (and free bar snacks) at Claridge's, tea (and cake) at Bill's Produce Store, late-night calls from friends in faraway time zones, black cabs, magic five-dollar rings and New York, New York.